John Ebnezar CBS Handbooks in Orthopedics and Fractures

SERIES

Orthopedic Problems of Different Ages

Adult Trauma

Volume III

- Injuries of Pelvis and Hip
- Injuries of Spine

John Ebnezar

- Holder of the **Guinness Book of World Records** for the most number of books written by an individual in a single year.
- Listed in the **India Book of Records** for the most number of books written by an individual.
- Recipient of the highest civilian awards of Karnataka, the **Rajyotsava Award 2010** and the **Kempegowda Award 2011**.
- Recipient of the **Best Citizen of India Award** by the International Publishing house.
- Former Vice-President, the Indian Orthopaedic Association
- President, Neuro-Spinal Surgeons Association of India (Karnataka)
- CEO, Parimala Health Care Services, A ISO 9001:2008 Hospital, Bilekahalli, Bannerghatta Road, Bangalore
- Ebnezar Orthopedic Center, Bilekahalli, Bannerghatta Road, Bangalore
- Dr John's Orthopedic Clinic, near Reliance Mart, Arakere, BG Road, Bangalore
- Chairman, the Physically Handicapped and Paraplegic Charitable Trust of Karnataka®
- Founder President, Geriatric Orthopedic Society
- Founder President, Orthopedic Authors Association and All India Medical Authors Association
- Chairman, Karnataka Orthopedic Academy®
- President, Bangalore Holistic Academy
- Chairman, Rakesh Cultural Academy
- President, Vaidya Kala Ranga, Bangalore
- Secretary, SK Educational Society®
- Former Senior Specialist, Victoria Hospital, Bangalore Medical College, Bangalore
- Former Assistant Professor in Orthopedics, Devaraj Urs Medical College, Kolar, Karnataka
- Postgraduate teacher, Bangalore Baptist Hospital, Airport Road, Bangalore

JOHN EBNEZAR CBS | Handbooks in
Orthopedics and Fractures

SERIES

Orthopedic Problems of Different Ages

Adult Trauma

VOLUME III

- Injuries of Pelvis and Hip
- Injuries of Spine

John Ebnezar

MBBS, D'Ortho, DNB (Ortho), MNAMS (Ortho), PhD (Yoga)
Sports Medicine (Australia), INOR Fellow (UK), DAc, DMT

Consulting Orthopedic and Spine Surgeon,
Holistic Orthopedic Expert, and Sports Specialist
Bangalore

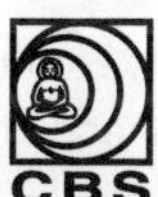

CBS Publishers & Distributors Pvt Ltd
New Delhi • Bengaluru • Pune • Kochi • Chennai

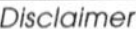

Disclaimer
Science and technology are constantly changing fields. New research and experience broaden the scope of information and knowledge. The author has tried his best in giving information available to him while preparing the material for this book. Although, all efforts have been made to ensure optimum accuracy of the material, yet it is quite possible some errors might have been left uncorrected. The publisher, printer and author will not be held responsible for any inadvertent errors or inaccuracies.

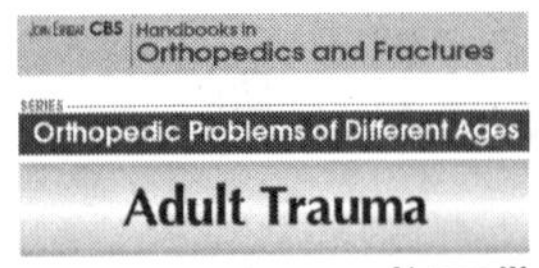

VOLUME III

ISBN: 978-81-239-2157-0

First Edition: 2012

Published by Satish Kumar Jain and produced by Vinod K. Jain for
CBS Publishers & Distributors Pvt Ltd
4819/XI Prahlad Street, 24 Ansari Road, Daryaganj
New Delhi 110 002, India.
Ph: 23289259, 23266861, 23266867
Fax: 011-23243014
Website: www.cbspd.com
e-mail: delhi@cbspd.com
cbspubs@airtelmail.in.

Branches

- Bengaluru: Seema House 2975, 17th Cross, K.R. Road, Banasankari 2nd Stage, Bengaluru 560 070, Karnataka
  Ph: +91-80-26771678/79 Fax: +91-80-26771680 e-mail: bangalore@cbspd.com
- Pune: Bhuruk Prestige, Sr. No. 52/12/2+1+3/2 Narhe, Haveli (Near Katraj-Dehu Road Bypass), Pune 411 051, Maharashtra
  Ph: 020-64704058, 64704059, 32392277 Fax: +91-020-24300160 e-mail: pune@cbspd.com
- Kochi: 36/14 Kalluvilakam, Lissie Hospital Road, Kochi 682 018, Kerala
  Ph: +91-484-4059061-65 Fax: +91-484-4059065 e-mail: cochin@cbspd.com
- Chennai: 20, West Park Road, Shenoy Nagar, Chennai 600 030, Tamil Nadu
  Ph: +91-44-26260666, 26208620 Fax: +91-44-45530020 email: chennai@cbspd.com

Printed at Magic International, Greater Noida (UP)

to

---

my mother
(late) Sampath Kumari
who taught me that life is more than self and
there is more joy in giving and sharing than taking

my wife
Dr Parimala

my lovely children
Rakesh and Priyanka
who are an epitome of love, sacrifice, encouragement
and inspiration

all my teachers
who made me what I am today

all my students
past and present

and

all my patients

Dr John Ebnezar

is a legendary name as a prolific orthopedic writer. No other orthopedic surgeon in the world has come anywhere close to him in the number of books he has written in his field. He is the first orthopedic surgeon in the world to be listed in the **Guinness Book of World Records** for the most number of books written by an individual in a single year. For the same feat his name has been listed in the **India Book of Records.** This book, like all his previous books, carries his flavor of simple and lucid writing, excellent language, beautiful illustrations and excellent presentation of the topics. This book is a part of the 100+ book series he has brought out in a single calendar year of 2012 on a wide array of orthopedic problems of public health importance. No other individual in the world has brought out these many books in one year and this is a world record attempt. With these books he aims to educate the reader and the public about these common orthopedic problems.

All his books have been accepted very well and he has a great fan following all over the world. He has been bestowed with as many as 32 international, national and state awards including Karnataka state's highest civilian award the **Rajyotsava Award 2010** and the **Kempegowda Award 2011,** apart from the **Best Citizen of India Award** given by the International Publishing House. He is the pioneer in holistic orthopedics and is credited for discovering a new method of treatment for the common orthopedic problems and has done PhD in arthritis from the world famous S-VYASA University, Bangalore. He is currently president of the Neuro-Spinal Surgeons Association of India (Karnataka), the former Vice-President of the Indian Orthopedic Association, and is the founder president of various orthopedic bodies.

Preface

This book is a part of the 100$^+$ book series

JOHN EBNEZAR CBS Handbooks in Orthopedics and Fractures

which deals with the orthopedic problems of public health importance. The purpose of these books is to educate and create awareness among the readers about various problems associated with orthopedics. Through this way the readers get to know all about various orthopedic problems directly from a specialist. This will help a reader immensely in getting the right knowledge as most of them depend on the internet and magazines which distort and misrepresent various pieces of information concerning health topics, leaving the readers confused and worse still improperly educated. This may harm more than helping them find solutions to their problems. The purpose of these books, therefore, is to educate the readers right in their quest for knowledge on the common health and associated problems.

The 100$^+$ book series has been brought out in a single calendar year.

This is a unique book, first of its kind that deals with the various common adult orthopedic injuries encountered in the adult population. This book gives an insight into various orthopedic problems peculiar to people in the adulthood, their causes, presentation, investigations, treatment, complications and their impact on the individual health and the society in general. This is the first ever book which exclusively deals with all the common orthopedic problems in the adults. Many of the patients were asking for a book on this topic so that they could understand all about the common orthopedic problems that are exclusively or more commonly seen in adults and the role they need to play in their prevention and treatment of these conditions.

Highlights of this book

- Simple and lucid language
- Good illustrations

- Good clinical photographs wherever necessary
- Relevant X-rays
- Short summaries
- Anecdotes
- Suggestions for self-help techniques for the adults

This book has ubiquitous utility and usage and can be useful to the orthopedic surgeons, postgraduate students in orthopedics, undergraduate medical students, doctors from all disciplines of medicine, physiotherapists, therapists practising alternative systems of medicine, rehabilitation specialists, and most importantly the common people. It is particularly useful to those unsung heroes who work in remote areas with minimum infrastructure. They can use this book as a ready-reckoner. Seldom will you find a book that covers such a wide spectrum of readers.

Knowing all about problems affecting the adult population creates an awareness and helps one to treat the problem thereby prevent the problems of old age from happening at the first place.

Please remember that this book is meant to educate and not substitute the role of a doctor. I advise the adult patients to see an orthopedic surgeon if they are suffering from any of the orthopedic problems and use this book to update your knowledge about the condition and practice simple self-help techniques apart from adhering to the do's and don'ts for each condition.

Constructive criticism and useful suggestions are invited to make the book more effective in its forthcoming editions.

John Ebnezar

Acknowledgments

This volume is a part of the 100^{+} book series brought out in a single calendar year. This was a huge and mammoth task attempted first time ever by an author and a publisher in the world. Such an herculean effort could not have been possible without the active involvement of those concerned in CBS Publishers & Distributors. I thank Mr Satish K Jain, Managing Director of CBS P&D, for agreeing to be a part of this world-record feat in bringing out this book in the Series. My special thanks to Mr YN Arjuna who showed special interest in this work and channelized his entire energy into this improbable feat. My special thanks to Mrs Ritu Chawla and her entire dedicated team who have toiled day and night to make this dream a reality. I thank members of the entire editorial–production team of CBS P&D who have worked hard behind the scenes to bring out this book.

My special thanks to Dr Yogitha for actively helping me in the compilation of all the books. I also thank all the staff members of my hospital who have helped me at various levels during the making of this book.

John Ebnezar

Contents

Preface *vii*

Section I: Injuries of Pelvis and Hip

1. Pelvic Injuries **3**

Fracture pelvis 3
Stability of the pelvis 3
Key and Conwell's classification 8
Tile's classification 9
Hemorrhage 16

2. Injuries of the Coccyx and Ribs **19**

Rib fractures 21
Principles of treatment 23
Conservative measures 23
Chest physiotherapy 23

3. Acetabular Fractures **24**

Epidemiology 25
Pathophysiology 26
Judet and Letournel classifications 27
Letournel classification 28
Transverse fractures 29
Radiological assessment of the acetabular fracture 31
Anteroposterior radiograph lines 31
CT scan 31
Transverse fractures 35
T-type fractures 37
Both-column fractures 38
Surgical approaches 42

4. Injuries Around the Hip Joint: Dislocations and Fracture Dislocations **44**

Posterior hip dislocations 48
Thompson and Epstein classifications 49
Pipkin types (Dislocation of the hip with fractures of the femoral head) 50

Goal of treatment 54
Allis method 55
Bigelow's method 55
Classical Watson-Jones method 56
Stimson's gravity method 57
Postreduction protocol 58
Indications for open reduction 59
Technique of open reduction 59
Postoperative treatment 60
Anterior dislocation of the hip 63
Epstein's classification 64
ABCDS method of reduction 66
Postreduction protocol 68
Delayed complications 68
Central dislocation of hip 69
Classification: Judet's types 69

5. Injuries Around the Hip—Fractures of Neck Femour 75

Upper or proximal femoral fractures 75
Fracture neck of femur 75
Vascular anatomy and its significance 77
Choices of implants for internal fixation 89
Cardinal points in internal fixation 90
Meyer's muscle pedicle graft 91
Thromboembolism 92
Osteotomy 94
Avascular necrosis 97
Trochanteric fracture 98
Choice of an implant 101

Section II: Injuries of Spine

6. Spinal Injuries 109

Incidence of spine injuries 113
Injuries of the cervical spine 113
Allen's classification of cervical spine fractures 116
Vital steps 122
Individual cervical fracture of interest 128
Burst fracture of C1 128
Odontoid process fracture 129
Hangman's fracture 129

7. Thoracic and Lumbosacral Spine Injuries 130

McAfee's classification—3-column classification 130
Modified Magerl classification (AO/ASIF) 132

8. Spnial Cord Injury 139

Clinical classification of neurological damage 139
Bedsore management 144
Bowel program 145
Cauda equina syndrome 147
Prognosis in spinal cord injuries 149

9. Peripheral Nerve Injury 151

Ulnar nerve injury 151
Causes of ulnar nerve injury 151
Claw hand 153
Treatment of ulnar nerve injury 157
Choice of surgery 158
Entrapment neuropathy 159
Radial nerve injury 160
Causes for radial nerve injury 160
Injury to sciatic nerve 167
Foot-drop 168
Causes of foot-drop 168
Treatment of early foot-drop 170
Meralgia paresthetica 173
Diagnostic test 173
Brachial plexus injuries 174
Supraclavicular lesion 175
Clinical assessment of brachial plexus injury 176
Surgical measures 178
Erb's palsy 179
Effects of the injury 179
Klumpke's paralysis 180
Axillary nerve injury 181
Relevant anatomy 181
Injury to the long thoracic nerve (Winging of the scapula) 182

Index 185

John Ebnezar **CBS** Handbooks in

Orthopedics and Fractures

TITLES IN THE SERIES

I Orthopedic Trauma

General Fractures

1 General Principles of Fractures and Dislocations
2 Fracture Treatment Methods
3 Fractures and their Complications
4 Atypical Fractures

Injuries of Upper Limb

5 Injuries of Shoulder
6 Injuries of Arm
7 Injuries of Elbow
8 Injuries of Forearm
9 Injuries of Wrist and Hand
10 Injuries of Distal Forearm and Wrist
11 Injuries of Hand
12 Injuries of Upper Limb

Injuries of Lower Limb

13 Injuries of Hip
14 Injuries of Femur
15 Injuries of Knee
16 Injuries of Knee and Leg
17 Injuries of Ankle and Leg
18 Injuries of Foot and Ankle
19 Injuries of Lower Limb

Injuries of Axial Skeleton

20 Injuries of Pelvis and Hip
21 Injuries of Spine
22 Injuries of Pelvis and Spine

23 Sports Injuries Volume I
24 Sports Injuries Volume II
25 Soft Tissue Problems in Orthopedics
26 Geriatric Trauma
27 Pediatric Trauma

II Orthopedic Disease

28 Congenital Orthopedic Problems
29 Developmental Orthopedic Problems

30 Metabolic Orthopedic Problems
31 Infective Orthopedic Problems
32 Disorders of Joints
33 Skeletal Tuberculosis
34 Inflammatory Orthopedic Problems
35 Degenerative Orthopedic Problems
36 Tumor Conditions in Orthopedics
37 Neuromuscular Disorders in Orthopedics

III Specific Orthopedic Problems

38 Orthopedic Problems of Spine
39 Orthopedic Problems of Neck
40 Orthopedic Problems of Hip
41 Orthopedic Problems of Knee
42 Orthopedic Problems of Foot
43 Orthopedic Problems of Shoulder
44 Orthopedic Problems of Elbow
45 Orthopedic Problems of Forearm
46 Orthopedic Problems of Wrist
47 Orthopedic Problems of Hand

IV Regional Orthopedic Problems

48 Regional Orthopedic Problems of Upper Limb
49 Regional Orthopedic Problems of Lower Limb
50 Regional Orthopedic Problems of Spine
51 Regional Orthopedic Problems of Hand

V Orthopedic Injuries and Surgeries

Upper Limb
52 Injuries and Surgeries of Humerus
53 Injuries and Surgeries of Forearm
54 Injuries and Surgeries of Hand and Wrist

Lower Limb
55 Injuries and Surgeries of Hip
56 Injuries and Surgeries of Femur
57 Injuries and Surgeries of Tibia
58 Injuries and Surgeries of Foot and Ankle

59 Common Surgeries of Spine
60 Interlocking Surgeries in Orthopedics
61 Arthroscopy
62 Arthroplasty

VI Practical Examination

63 Long Cases in Practical Orthopedic Examination
64 Short Cases in Practical Orthopedic Examination
65 Viva Voce Examination: Typical X-rays
66 Viva Voce Examination: Instruments and Implants
67 Viva Voce Examination: Prosthetics, Orthotics and Traction
68 Viva Voce Examination: Ward Rounds, Specimen, Slides and Spotters
69 Viva Voce Examination: Common Orthopedic Surgeries
70 Viva Voce in Practical Orthopedic Examination VOLUME I
71 Viva Voce in Practical Orthopedic Examination VOLUME II

VII Orthopedic Problems of Different Ages

72 Pediatric Orthopedic Problems
73 Adult Orthopedic Problems VOLUME I
74 Adult Orthopedic Problems VOLUME II
75 Adult Trauma VOLUME I
76 Adult Trauma VOLUME II
77 Adult Trauma VOLUME III
78 Geriatric Orthopedic Problems
79 Orthopedic Problems in Women VOLUME I
80 Orthopedic Problems in Women VOLUME II
81 Orthopedic Problems in Women VOLUME III
82 Orthopedic Problems of Public Health Importance VOLUME I
83 Orthopedic Problems of Public Health Importance VOLUME II
84 Orthopedic Problems of Public Health Importance VOLUME III
85 Orthopedic Problems of Public Health Importance VOLUME IV

VIII Common Orthopedic Problems

86 Low Backache
87 Osteoarthritis
88 Common Neck Pain
89 Common Upper Limb Pain

90 Osteoporosis
91 Foot Pain
92 Rheumatoid Arthritis

IX Yoga Therapy in Common Orthopedic Problems

93 Yoga Therapy for Low Backache
94 Yoga Therapy for Knee Pain
95 Yoga Therapy for Neck Pain
96 Yoga Therapy for Osteoporosis
97 Yoga Therapy for Frozen Shoulder
98 Yoga Therapy for Tennis Elbow
99 Yoga Therapy for Carpal Tunnel Syndrome
100 Yoga Therapy for Heel Pain
101 Yoga Therapy for Repetitive Stress Injury
102 Yoga Therapy for Rheumatoid Arthritis
103 Yoga Therapy for Fractures

Section I

Injuries of Pelvis and Hip

Pelvic Injuries

This book deals with injuries of axial skeleton in adults

Brief anatomy of pelvis

The pelvis is made up of two innominate bones, a portion of spine and sacrum (Fig. 1.1). The innominate bone is formed by fusion of three separate bones, the ilium, ischium and pubis. Ilium forms the superior part, the ischium the posteroinferior part and the pubis the anteroinferior part. These three bones meet to form the acetabulum. Anteriorly it is connected by a strong minimally mobile fibrocartilaginous joint called the pubic symphysis. Posteriorly it articulates with the sacrum through the almost immobile sacroiliac joint. It derives its stability in the posterior aspect from the sacroiliac (SI) and the sacrospinous ligament complex, anteriorly by the pubic symphysis and inferiorly by the muscles and ligaments forming the pelvic floor and perineum. Its main functions are

- To transmit the forces from the spine to the lower limbs and vice versa.
- In the standing position, it transmits the weight through the ilium and in the sitting position through the ischium.
- It gives attachment to the muscles helping in posture and locomotion.
- It protects the vital genitourinary system and lower abdominal viscera.

FRACTURE PELVIS

Stability of the Pelvis

Stability of the pelvis depends on both bony and ligamentous structures. Anterior portion of the pelvic ring neither participates in normal weight bearing nor is it essential for maintenance of pelvic stability. The posterior arch is formed by the sacrum, SI joints and ilia and is the weight-bearing portion of the pelvis. The posterosuperior SI ligaments provide most of the ligamentous stability of the SI joints.

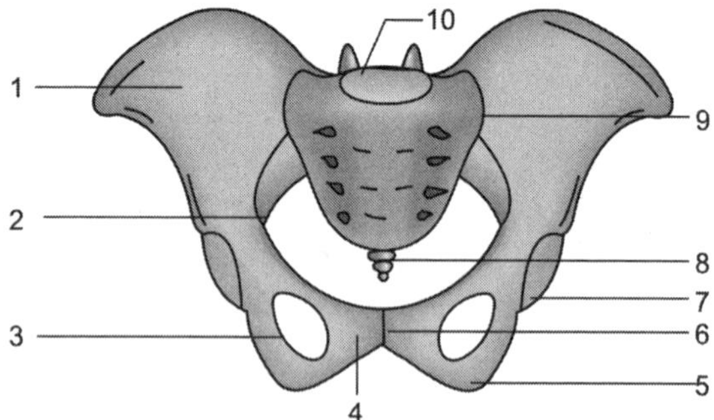

Fig. 1.1: Anatomy of pelvis: (1) Ilium, (2) Arcuate line, (3) Obturator foramen, (4) Pubis, (5) Ischium, (6) Pubic symphysis, (7) Acetabulum, (8) Coccyx, (9) Sacroiliac, (10) Sacrum

Stable Pelvic Fracture

These fractures do not involve the pelvic ring and they are minimally displaced.

Unstable Pelvic Fracture

They involve the pelvic ring and are widely displaced. Pelvic fractures pose a problem different from others. Here the emphasis is on recognition of potential complications associated with these fractures, the notable ones being injuries to the major vessels and nerves of the pelvis and major viscera like intestines, bladder and the urethra, severe intrapelvic hemorrhage from fracture of pelvic ring. Mortality from pelvic fracture varies from 10–50 percent. Proper fracture management decreases the blood loss and controls the hemorrhage. A to F management as proposed by McMurtry in multiple trauma patients is important in management of the pelvic fractures.

History

Pelvic fractures usually occur due to high-velocity trauma following a road traffic accident (RTA) or due to fall from a height.

Vital practice points

A to F management of McMurtry

A. Airway management
B. Blood and fluid replacement
C. Central nervous system management
D. Digestive system management
E. Excretory system management
F. Fracture management.

The relative incidences are as follows:

- RTA—80.7 percent.
- Fall—16.1 percent.
- Compression fracture—rest.

Mechanism of Injury

There are four mechanisms by which pelvic ring fractures are produced:

- Lateral compression (Fig. 1.2A).
- Anteroposterior compression (Fig. 1.2B).
- Vertical shears forces.
- Inferior forces, e.g. fall on buttocks.

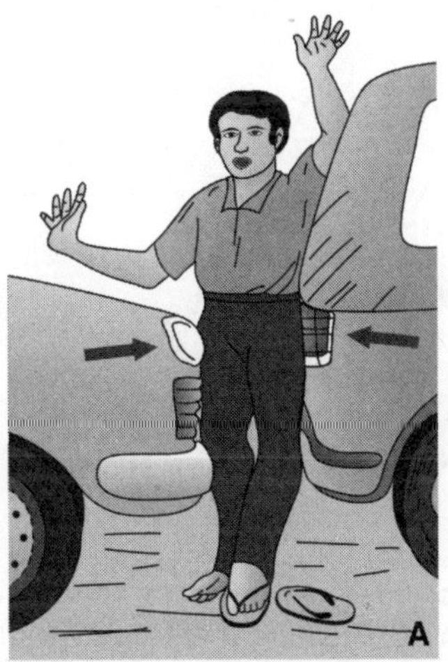

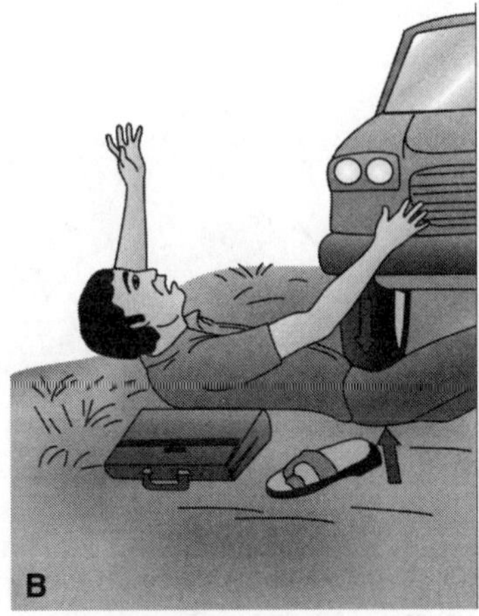

Figs 1.2A and B: Mechanism of pelvic fractures in RTA: (A) Lateral compression, (B) Anteroposterior compression

The first two mechanisms are common in RTA and may cause stable or unstable fractures. Vertical shear forces are due to fall from a height and will cause grossly unstable fractures.

Fortunately, most pelvic fractures are stable and respond to nonoperative treatment. Unstable fractures need manipulative reduction and stabilization by external fixators and sometimes by internal fixation. A proper evaluation of the fracture by radiograph and CT scan helps to determine the best course of management.

Classification

Broadly speaking, the pelvic fractures can be placed under two categories.

Fractures not Affecting the Integrity of the Pelvic Ring

Direct blow fractures, which are commonly seen in iliac bone and avulsion fractures frequently encountered in the young, come under this group. Avulsion fractures are commonly seen in anterosuperior and inferior iliac spines and ischial tuberosity (Fig. 1.3).

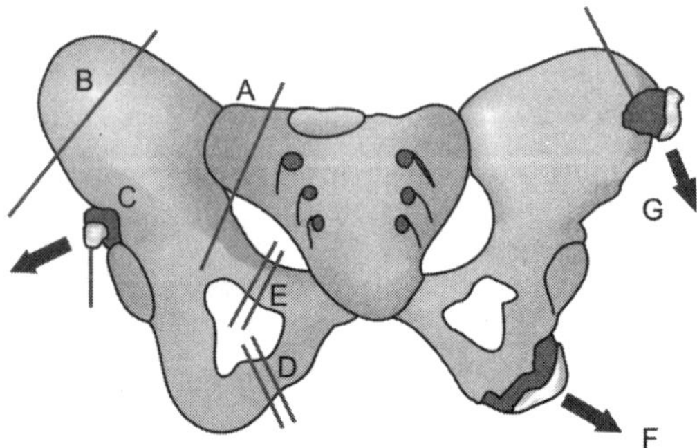

Fig. 1.3: Avulsion fractures and fractures of individual bones not affecting the pelvic ring: (A) Fracture of the sacrum, (B) Fracture of the iliac wing, (C) Aavulsion fracture of anteroinferior iliac spine, (D) Inferior rami fracture, (E) Superior ramus fracture, (F) Avulsion fracture of ischial tuberosity, and (G) Avulsion fracture of anterosuperior iliac spine

Fractures Affecting the Integrity of the Pelvic Ring

These are single or double break fractures in the pelvic ring and could be stable or unstable. A stable fracture is one, which resists displacing forces (Fig. 1.4). Obviously, fractures which cannot resist usual forces, are called unstable fractures and these pose a major therapeutic challenge (Fig. 1.5).

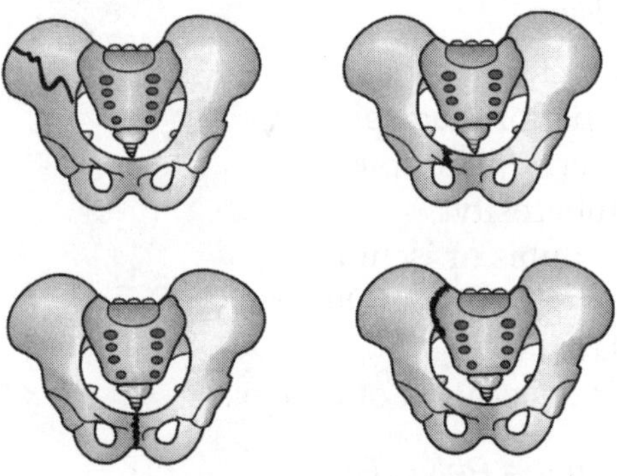

Fig. 1.4: Stable pelvic fractures

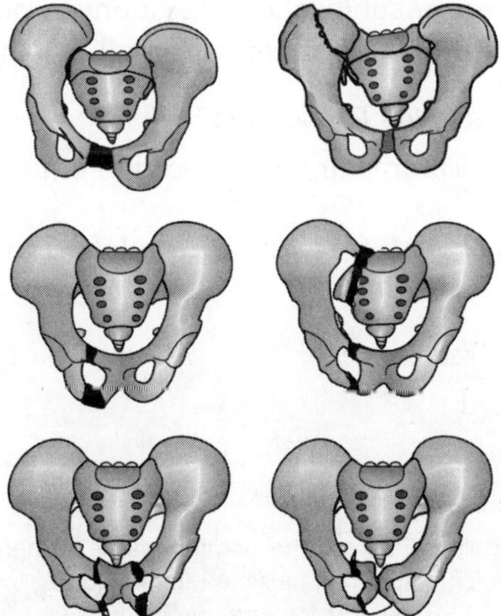

Fig. 1.5: Unstable pelvic fractures

Many classifications have been proposed for pelvic fractures. Key and Conwell's classification is by far the simplest and commonly used classification. It has prognostic importance too.

Key and Conwell's Classification

Fracture of Individual Bones without a Break in the Pelvic Ring

- Avulsion fracture of the
  - anterosuperior iliac spine
  - anteroinferior iliac spine
  - ischial tuberosity.
- Fracture of pubis or ischium.
- Fracture wing of ilium (Duverney).
- Fracture sacrum.
- Fracture or dislocation of coccyx.

Single Break in the Pelvic Ring

- Fracture of both ipsilateral rami.
- Fracture near or subluxation of symphysis pubis.
- Fracture near or subluxation of sacroiliac joints.

Double Breaks in the Pelvic Ring

- Double vertical fracture or dislocation of pubis *(Straddle fracture).*
- Double vertical fracture or dislocation of pelvis *(Malgaigne's fracture).*

Acetabulum Fractures

- Undisplaced.
- Displaced.

Relative incidence

- Fracture pubic bones are the commonest > 69 percent. Single ramus more common than multiple rami fracture.
- Malgaigne—11.8 percent fracture.
- Multiple crush injuries—10.8 percent fracture.
- Wing of ilium—5.4 percent fracture.

Tile's Classification

This is a mechanical classification based on the injury forces.

Type A	Stable.
Type A1	Fracture pelvis not involving ring.
Type A2	Stable, but minimally displaced.
Type B	Rotationally unstable but vertically stable.
Type B1	Open book injury.
Type B2	Lateral compression—Ipsilateral.
Type B3	Lateral compression—Contralateral. (Bucket handle).
Type C	Rotationally and vertically unstable.
Type C1	Rotationally and vertically unstable.
Type C2	Bilateral.
Type C3	Associated with acetabular fractures.

Murel-Lavallee Lesion

This is a closed degloving injury with traumatic shearing of skin from deep fascia. It leaves a large dead space prone for infection.

Treatment consists of debridement and primary closure of soft tissues.

Clinical Features

Symptoms

The patient most often gives a history of high-velocity trauma and usually presents in a state of hypovolaemic shock. Features of intra-abdominal injuries and genitourinary injuries are frequently present.

Clinical Signs

The patient may present with all signs of shock. Tenderness over the fracture site and one has to look for three important signs described by Milch.

Clinical Tests

Compression test: When a compressive force is applied through the two iliac bones, the patient complains of pain in pelvic fracture (Fig. 1.6A).

Quick facts

Look for the signs of shock in pelvic fracture

- Pale look
- Cold nose
- Sweating
- Tachycardia
- Hypotension
- Cold and clammy skin
- Unconsciousness.

Clinical points: Milch signs

Destot's sign: Large hematoma above inguinal ligament or scrotum.
Roux's sign: Distance from greater trochanter to pubic spine is ↑ on affected side.
Earle's sign: On per rectal examination, the bony prominence or a large hematoma can be palpated.

Distraction test: When distraction force is applied to the two iliac bones at the anterosuperior iliac spine, the patient complains of pain (Fig. 1.6B).

Direct pressure test: Direct pressure over the symphysis pubis elicits pain (Fig. 1.6C).

Following this, an examination for abdomen and pelvis injuries is carried out and next urethral catheterization or urethrogram is done.

Investigations

Radiography

Different radiographic views are recommended to study the fracture configuration, displacements, etc. (Figs 1.7A to C) in pelvic fractures

- Plain AP view.
- Oblique view—45° oblique projections.
- Internal and external rotation view.
- Inlet view—40° caudad view.
- Outlet view—40° cephalad view.

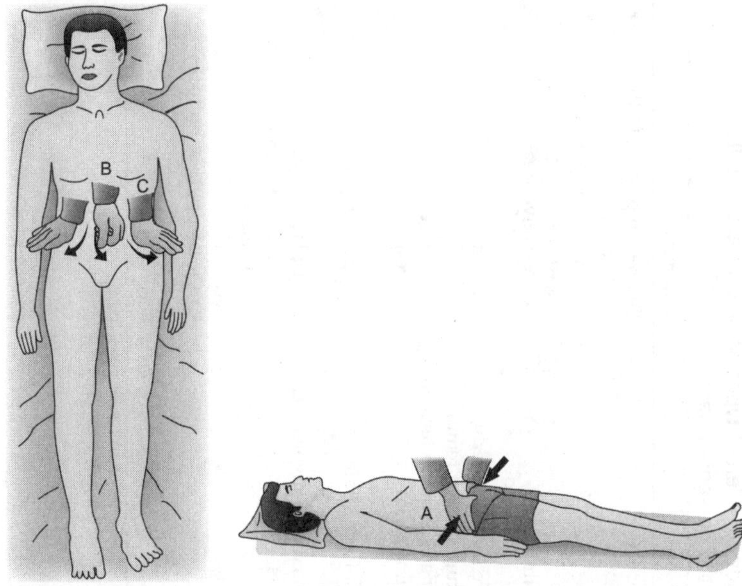

Fig. 1.6: (A) Compression test in pelvic fractures, (B) Direct pressure test, (C) Distraction test

CT Scan

Further radiographic studies include CT scans and 3-dimensional imaging. This is the gold standard in the evaluation of pelvic fractures.

Management

One should remember that pelvic fractures are usually due to high-velocity trauma and is associated with multiple fractures and multiple system injuries. Resuscitation and correction of hypovolemic shock takes precedence over the management of fracture *per se*. Nevertheless, once the general condition is stabilized attention should be given to treat the fracture, which will prevent further blood loss and damage to visceral organs.

Different types of pelvic fractures, their clinical features and treatment are listed in the Table 1.1.

Table 1.1: Key and Conwell's types: A comparative study of different types of pelvic fractures, their clinical features and treatment is presented here

Sl. No.	*Type of pelvic fracture*	*Clinical features*	*Treatment*
Type I	• Avulsion of anterosuperior iliac spine	Pain on trying to flex and abduct the thigh	Bed rest, hip spica, ORIF rarely done
	• Avulsion of anteroinferior iliac spine	Rare	Rest with hip flexed for 2–3 weeks
	• Avulsion of ischial tuberosity	Flexion of thigh with knee in flexion - pain	Conservative treatment
	• Single ramus fracture of pubis or ischium	Commonest fracture seen in elderly, confused with fracture neck of femur	Bed rest
	• Fracture body of ischium	Pain when hamstrings are put in tension	Bed rest
	• Stress fracture pubis or ischium fracture	Can occur in last trimester of pregnancy	Bed rest
	• Fracture iliac wing (6%)	Lateral compression force - pain Walking is painful	Strapping of pelvis
	• Fracture sacrum	Neurological deficits due to involvement of higher sacral roots	Undisplaced fracture; bed rest In neurological lesions posterior sacral laminectomy is done
	• Fracture coccyx	Fall in sitting position	Bed rest Cross-strapping of buttocks In severe disability, coccygectomy

Contd.

Table 1.1: Key and Conwell's types: A comparative study of different types of pelvic fractures, their clinical features and treatment is presented here *(Contd.)*

Sl. No.	*Type of pelvic fracture*	*Clinical features*	*Treatment*
Type II	• Fracture of two rami ipsilateral	Flexion, abduction and external rotation (FABER) test is positive. This fracture is common **FABER—Flexion abduction and external rotation**	Bed rest; bucks traction
	• Fracture or subluxation near symphysis pubis	Tenderness over symphysis pubis + palpable gap + injury to genitourinary tract common.	Circumferential strapping
	• Fracture or subluxation near SI joint	FABER test is positive Straight leg raising test is painful	Symptomatic treatment and bed rest, pelvic sling, belt
Type III	• Double vertical fracture **(Straddle fracture)**	Urethral injury—20% Abdominal injury—38%	Symptomatic treatment, bed rest, etc.
	• **Malgaigne's fracture** (Ipsilateral pubic rami fracture with ipsilateral SI joint (dislocation)	Shortening, external rotation deformity, limb shortening, umbilicus displaced	Postural reduction + traction + pelvic slings
	• Severe multiple fracture of pelvis	Associated with severe visceral damage	• In compound fracture external fixators preferred • Open reduction and internal fixation if associated with multiple system injuries • Rest in bed with sand bags, pelvic slings and traction
Type IV	Fracture acetabulum	Could be displaced or undisplaced, could be a rim fracture or central floor fracture	Skeletal traction through the greater trochanter

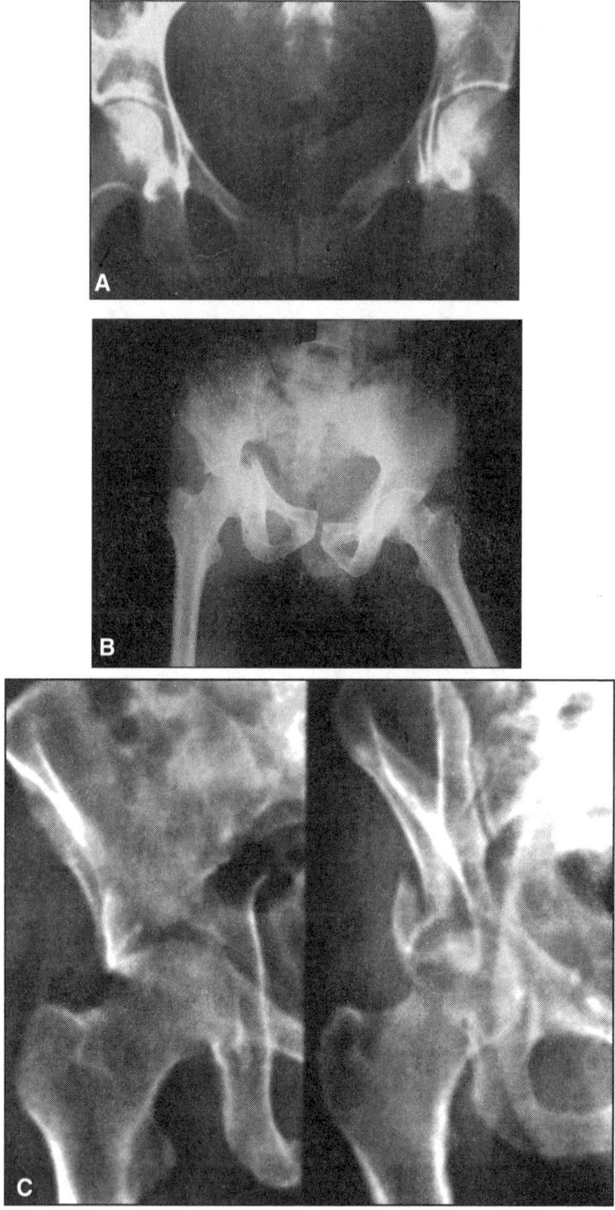

Figs 1.7A to C: (A) Superior ramus fracture, (B) Fracture acetabulum and separation of symphysis, (C) Pelvic floor fracture

Treatment points

Three main pitfalls in the treatment of pelvic fracture

- Treating only fracture overlooking visceral injuries.
- Over treating a stable fracture.
- Treating an unstable fracture.

Treatment Methods

Initial treatment is carried out as follows:

- Resuscitation and other general measures, to improve the general condition of the patient.
- Blood transfusion and other medical and surgical emergency measures are carried out.

Avulsion fractures: Conservative treatment like bed rest, traction, physiotherapy, etc. gives good results. They rarely need surgery.

Undisplaced fractures: Respond to bed rest, traction, pelvic slings (Fig. 1.8), nonsteroidal anti-inflammatory drugs (NSAIDs), etc.

Displaced fractures: Reduction by lateral compression methods as described by Watson Jones is very helpful. Retention is by spica cast, canvas sling or external fixators.

Role of external and internal fixators: The above methods usually suffice, but the fractures associated with multiple

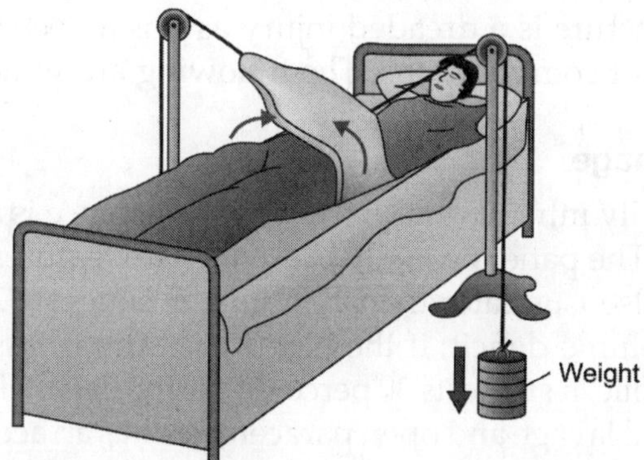

Fig. 1.8: Pelvic sling as a mainstay of conservative treatment in fracture pelvis

system injuries need to be stabilized either by external fixators or by open reduction and internal fixation (ORIF) (Fig. 1.9). These two methods have the following advantages:

- Gives firm stability.
- Helps early mobilization.
- Reduces period of bed rest.
- Helps early control of osseous bleeding.

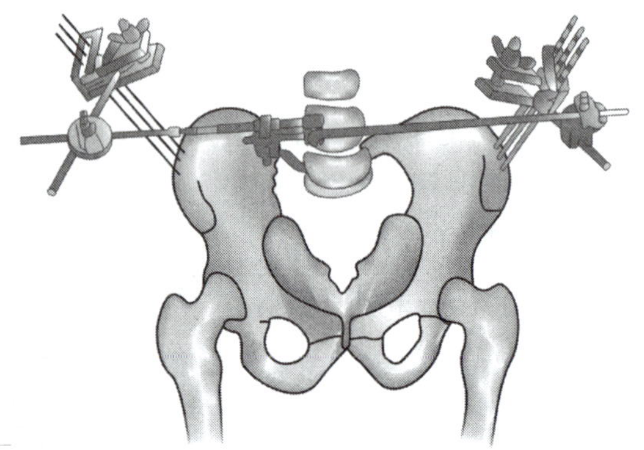

Fig. 1.9: Treatment by external fixation methods in pelvic fractures

Complications

Pelvic fracture is a dreaded injury as it is associated with a plethora of complications. The following are some of them.

Hemorrhage

It is usually intra-abdominal and the incidence is around 20 percent. The patient usually presents with features of shock. If the pulse is greater than 100/min, it suggests 20 percent blood volume deficit; if the blood pressure is less than 100 mm systolic, it suggests 30 percent volume deficit. Diagnostic peritoneal lavage and open paracentesis has an accuracy rate of 98 percent in intra-abdominal injuries. CT scan is also sensitive and specific.

Treatment is by laparotomy and is indicated if there is continuing blood loss, visceral perforation, expanding palpable suprapubic hematoma.

Injuries of Lower Urinary Tract

Rupture of urethra and rupture of urinary bladder are the common lower urinary tract injuries frequently seen in separation of pubic symphysis and fracture pubic rami. It has an average incidence of 13 percent. The dictum is *All pelvic fractures must be assumed to have urinary tract injuries until proved otherwise.*

Presence of hematuria is not pathognomonic, but its presence calls for three radiographic studies like retrograde urethrogram, cystogram and IVP. Rupture of anterior urethra is seen in straddle fractures and is not very common. Rupture of posterior urethra is relatively more common and is limited to male. Suprapubic cystostomy, direct repair, railroad repair, urethroplasties are some of the treatment methods.

Bladder injuries are seen in 4 percent of the cases and are associated with symphysis pubis injuries and rami fracture. Eighty percent injuries are extra peritoneal and calls for direct surgical intervention as quickly as possible.

Other Injuries

Testicular injuries and vaginal lacerations, bowel and rectal injuries and urethral injuries are all common and require immediate surgical intervention.

Other Complications

Loss of reduction, sepsis, thrombophlebitis, delayed union, nonunion, post-traumatic arthritis, fat embolism, major arterial injuries, abdominal wall injury, neurological injuries usually L5, S1 roots due to sacral fracture are the other common complications.

Recap

Pelvic fractures

- A fracture feared for its complications.
- RTA accounts for 80 percent of cases.
- Fracture broadly classified into not affecting and affecting integrity of the pelvic ring.
- Fracture pubic rami, usually single, is the commonest pelvic fracture (69%).
- Usual presentation is hypovolemic shock.
- Correction of hypovolemia and other general measures takes precedence over fracture management.
- Conservative treatment usually gives good results.
- External and internal fixation is done for specific indications.
- Intra-abdominal and genitourinary injuries are common possibilities and need early recognition and prompt treatment.
- Mortality is 20 percent.

Note: Mortality in closed pelvic fractures is 10–30 percent and open fractures are 40–50 percent.

Quick facts: Interesting pelvic fractures

Straddle fracture: Double vertical fractures of pubic-rami.
Malgaigni's fracture: Ipsilateral pubic-rami fracture and SI joint dislocation.
Bucket handle fracture: Pubic-rami fracture with contralateral SI joint dislocation.
Open back fractures: Disruption of the pubic-symphysis or rami fracture and external rotation of the hemipelvis over an intact posterior SI joints.

2

Injuries of the Coccyx and Ribs

INJURY TO THE COCCYX

These are relatively rare injuries, but could be quite troublesome to the patients. This can lead to the development of coccydynia, which is described as a chronic pain in the coccyx.

Mechanism of Injury

It is due to a direct fall on the buttocks (Fig. 2.1). It can also result from seat injuries while driving two wheelers or four wheelers. Of late constant pressure due to prolonged sitting as in the case of computer professionals can give rise to coccydynia.

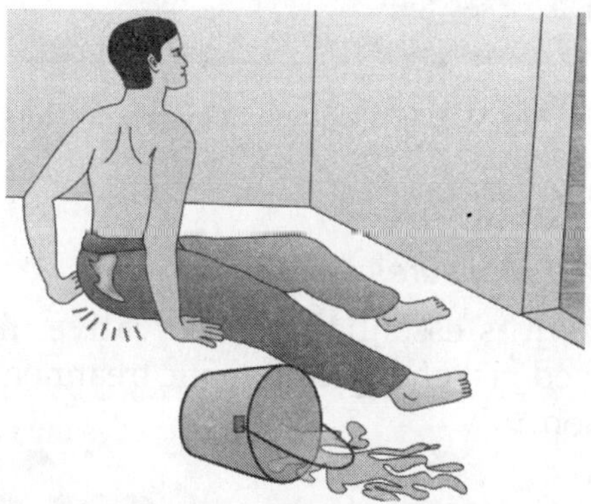

Fig. 2.1: Mechanism of injury in coccyx fractures

Clinical Features

The patient usually complains of pain in the buttocks and is unable to sit comfortably. Due to the development of coccydynia the pain may become chronic. The patient also complains of difficulty in traveling and altered sitting postures due to the pain.

Investigations

Plain X-ray of the coccyx especially the lateral view helps to make the diagnosis (Fig. 2.2). However, it is difficult to position the patient for the X-rays. MRI of the sacrococcygeal region is a better option.

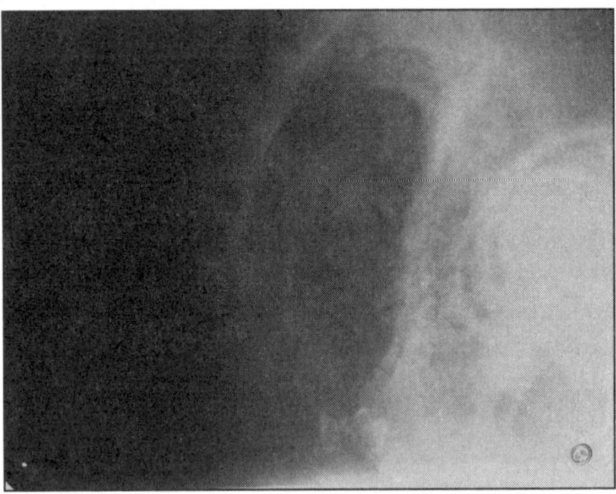

Fig. 2.2: Radiograph of coccyx fracture

Treatment

Conservative Measures

The treatment is essentially conservative in nature with periods of bed rest and symptomatic treatment for pain and inflammation.

Physiotherapy Management

Consists of the following steps:

- To relieve pain, thermotherapy likes ultrasound and TENS.
- To relieve prolonged pressure on the buttocks, sitting on a ring cushion and sitting on alternate buttocks is advised.
- Isometric exercises to the glutei maximus muscle in sitting, lying and prone positions are advisable.
- *Sitz bath helps to relieve pain.

Note: These injuries are difficult to tackle.

Reasons

- Due to the position of coccyx, which is deep and covered by thick muscles on either side?
- Due to the pressure from sitting. Hence, long sitting posture needs to be controlled.

Injection Therapy

If the pain is unrelieved by the usual conservative and physiotherapy measures, injection therapy consisting of a mixture of local steroids (Depomedorol, Kenacort, etc.) and xylocaine gives excellent relief of pain.

Surgical Excision of the Coccyx

In extreme situations if all the above measures fail then surgical removal of the coccyx may be considered.

RIB FRACTURES

These are relatively rare injuries and are usually due to direct trauma. The rib usually breaks at the angle, which is a point of maximum convexity (Fig. 2.3).

Clinical Features

The patient complains of pain in the affected region and has difficulty in breathing. He also complains of inability to sleep

---

*Sitz bath—this consists of sitting in a shallow tub of warm water. Commonly advocated in Piles patients after surgery.

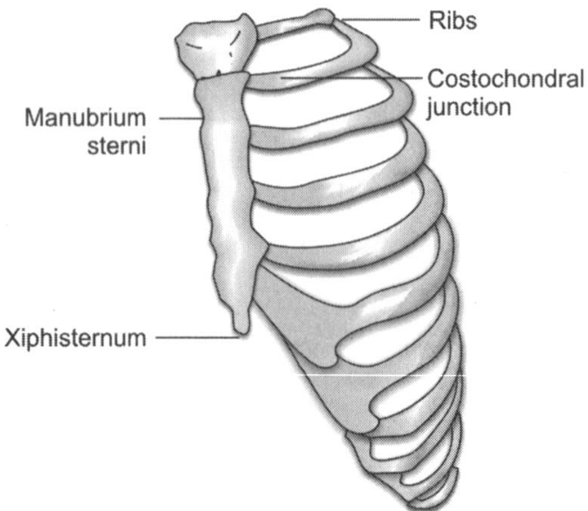

Fig. 2.3: Anatomical features of the ribs

on the affected side or lift weights and has difficulty in traveling or carrying out his day-to-day activities.

Radiology

Plain X-ray of the chest helps to detect the rib fractures with reasonable accuracy (Fig. 2.4).

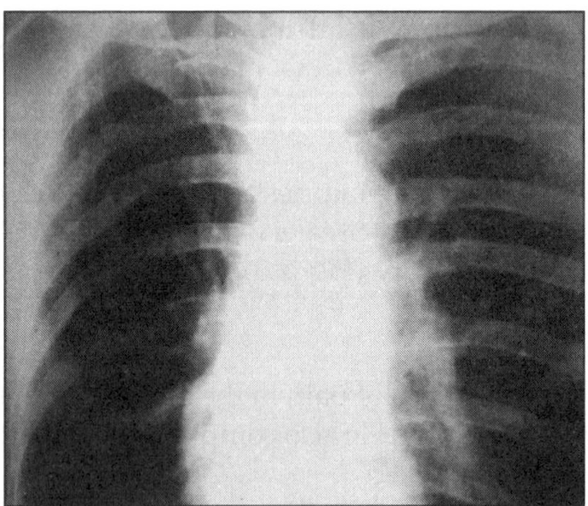

Fig. 2.4: Malunited right 2nd to 4th rib fractures

Principles of Treatment

It is essentially conservative. Intercostal muscles provide natural immobilization to the fractured ribs and hence no aggressive management is required.

Conservative Measures

Strapping (Fig. 2.5), ultrasound or TENS, etc. are effective in reducing the pain. Occasionally, a local infiltration of hydrocortisone helps. Very rarely, the fracture fragments may pierce the pleura causing pneumothorax, hemothorax, etc. These are dangerous injuries and needs to be managed aggressively.

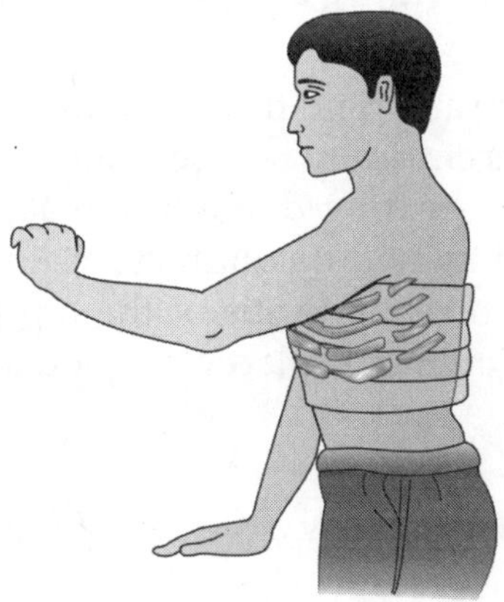

Fig. 2.5: Strapping method for treatment of fracture ribs

Chest Physiotherapy

This essentially consists of deep breathing exercises, which are progressively made more vigorous to improve the mobility of the thorax.

3 Acetabular Fractures

Introduction

This is an injury in young adults and is due to high-velocity RTAs and trauma. They are most of the times associated with other life-threatening injuries due to the high-velocity injuries.

Anatomic reduction and rigid fixation of the fracture, with the femoral head concentrically reduced under an adequate portion of the weight-bearing dome of the acetabulum, is the treatment goal in these difficult fractures for fear of the development of secondary arthritis of the hip joint due to joint incongruity following displaced acetabular fractures.

Relevant Anatomy

- The acetabulum is formed by a portion of the innominate bone.
- It lies at the point where the ilium, ischium, and pubis are joined by the triradiate cartilage, which later fuses to form the innominate bone. The innominate bone is irregular in shape and has differing thickness in cross section in different areas.
- The acetabulum is enclosed by the anterior and the posterior columns like the 2 limbs of an inverted Y, as shown in the Figs 3.1 to 3.3.

  The anterior column comprises of

  - The anterior border of the iliac wing,
  - The entire pelvic brim,

– The anterior wall of the acetabulum,
– The superior pubic ramus.

The posterior column comprises of

– The ischial portion of the bone,
– Including the greater and lesser sciatic notch,
– The posterior wall of the acetabulum,
– The majority of the quadrilateral surface, and
– The ischial tuberosity
– The roof of the acetabulum is the thick, weight bearing portion, and forms a separate fragment in bi-columnar fractures.
– The thin quadrilateral plate forms the medial wall or the floor of the acetabulum.

Epidemiology

- Incidence of acetabular fractures 24%.
- Admission rate for pelvic and acetabular fractures 0.5–7.5%.

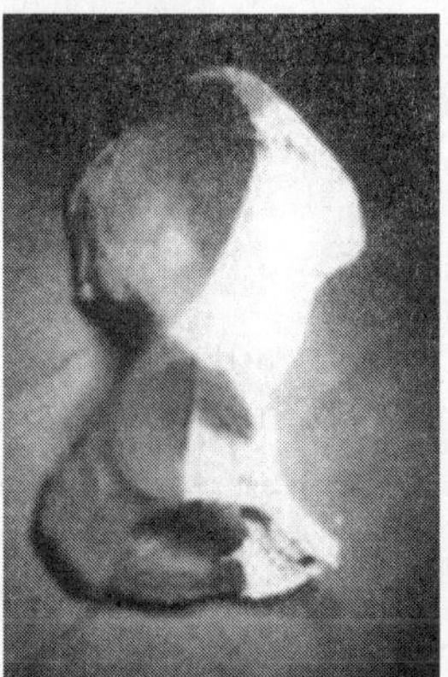

Fig. 3.1: Columns of the acetabulum, anteroposterior view. The white area is the anterior column, the red area is the posterior column, and the purple area is the tie beam (inferior pubic ramus)

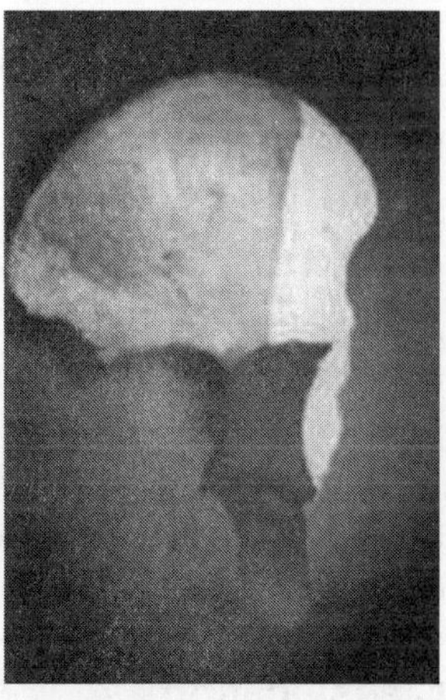

Fig. 3.2: Columns of the acetabulum, iliac view

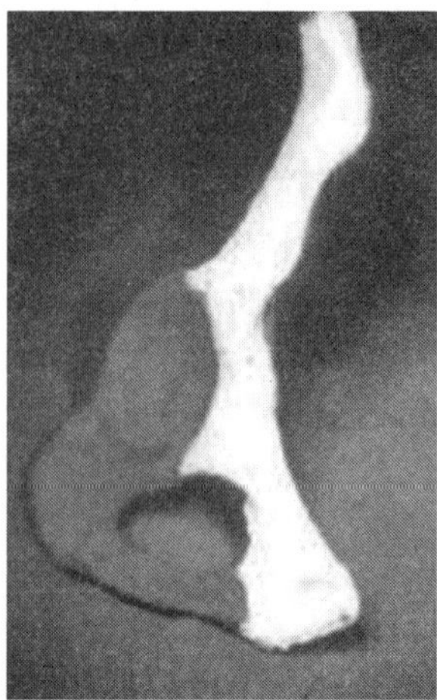

Fig. 3.3: Columns of the acetabulum, obturator view

- Approximately 5–10% of pediatric pelvic injuries involve the acetabulum.

Etiology

Acetabulum fractures usually occur as a result of high-velocity trauma, such as vehicular accidents or falls from heights.

Pathophysiology

Fractures of the acetabulum occur as a result of the force exerted through the head of the femur to the acetabulum.

The femoral head acts like a hammer and is the last link in the chain of forces transmitted from the greater trochanter, knee, or foot to the acetabulum.

The position of the femur at the time of impact and the direction of the force determine the type and displacement of the fracture.

Classification

For the purposes of classification of fracture patterns, the acetabulum is divided into (Fig. 3.4).

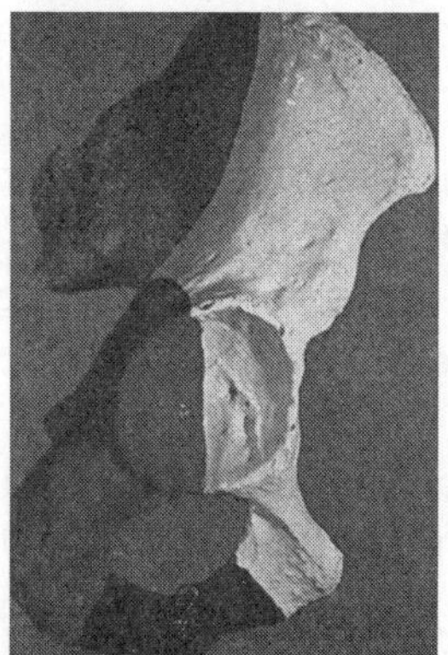

Fig. 3.4: The anterior and posterior columns

- Anterior column (Larger)
- Posterior column.

I. Judet and Letournel Classifications

They classify acetabular fractures according to the fracture morphology as elementary fracture pattern.

Posterior wall fractures: These fractures typically involve

- The rim of the acetabulum.
- A portion of the retroacetabular surface.
- A variable segment of the articular cartilage.
- The articular cartilage may also be impacted.

Note: Impacted articular cartilage should be diagnosed preoperatively on CT scan, as these impacted fragments require elevation at the time of surgery.

Extended posterior wall fractures can involve the entire retroacetabular surface and include a portion of the greater or lesser sciatic notch, the ischial tuberosity, or both.

The ilioischial line, however, remains intact on the anteroposterior (AP) view.

Posterior column fractures: These fractures include

- The ischial portion of the bone.

- The entire retroacetabular surface is displaced with the posterior column.
- As the vertical line separating the anterior column from the posterior column traverses inferiorly, it most commonly enters the obturator foramen.
- An associated fracture of the inferior pubic ramus is present.
- Sometimes, the fracture line traverses just posterior to the obturator foramen, splitting the ischial tuberosity.
- The ilioischial line typically is displaced and disassociated from the teardrop.
- However, when a large portion of the quadrilateral surface remains intact with the posterior column, the teardrop and a portion of the pelvic brim displace with the posterior column.

Anterior wall fractures: These fractures are uncommon injuries and often occur in conjunction with anterior dislocations.

Anterior column fractures: Low fractures involve

- Only the superior ramus and pubic portion of the acetabulum.
- High fractures can involve the entire anterior border of the innominate bone.
- The pelvic brim and iliopectineal line are displaced.
- Medial translation of the entire roof or a portion of the roof is typical of displacement of a high or intermediate anterior column fracture.

II. Letournel Classification

The most widely used classification of acetabular fractures is the Letournel classification, which is a modification of the 1964 Judet anatomic classification. Letournel's system classifies acetabular fractures into 10 major fracture patterns, which consist of 5 simple patterns and 5 complex patterns (Fig. 3.5)

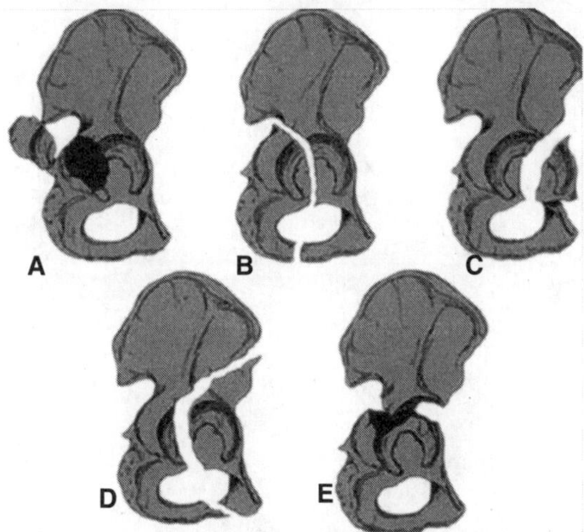

Figs 3.5A to E: Simple fracture patterns

The 5 simple patterns (Figs 3.5A to E)
- Posterior wall fractures (A)
- Posterior column fractures (B)
- Anterior wall fractures (C)
- Anterior column fractures (D)
- Transverse acetabular fractures (E)

The 5 complex patterns (Figs 3.6A to E)
- Posterior column with a posterior wall fracture (A)
- Transverse with a posterior wall fracture (B)
- T-type fracture (C)
- Anterior column with a posterior hemitransverse fracture (D)
- Both-column fracture (E)

TRANSVERSE FRACTURES

These fractures divide the innominate bone into 2 portions.
- A horizontally displaced fracture line crosses the acetabulum at a variable level.
- The innominate bone is then divided into a superior part and a lower part.

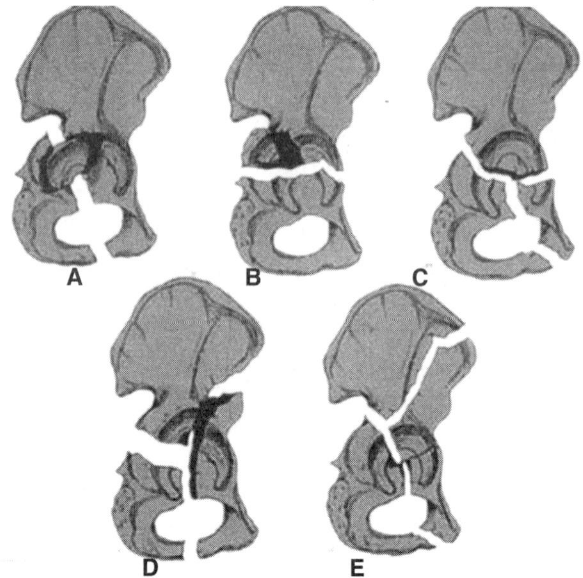

Figs 3.6A to E: The 5 complex fracture patterns

- The superior part is composed of the iliac wing and a portion of the roof of the acetabulum.
- The lower part of the bone, the ischiopubic segment, is composed of an intact obturator foramen with the anterior and posterior walls of the acetabulum.

  Letournel subclassified transverse fractures as follows
  - *Transtectal:* Here the transverse fracture line crosses the superior acetabular articular surface
  - *Juxtatectal:* Here the transverse fracture line crosses at the junction of the superior acetabular articular surface and superior cotyloid fossa
  - *Infratectal:* Here the transverse fracture line crosses through the cotyloid fossa.

III. The AO Classification

- *Type A fractures:* Involving either a single wall or column (anterior or posterior).

- *Type B fractures:* Include both anterior and posterior columns but not bicolumnar fractures (transverse, T-shaped, anterior with posterior hemitransverse type injuries)
- *Type C fractures:* Bicolumnar fractures, with the roof as a separate fragment.

RADIOLOGICAL ASSESSMENT OF THE ACETABULAR FRACTURE

Anteroposterior Radiograph Lines

On anteroposterior (AP) radiographs of the acetabulum, 6 major lines should be considered (Fig. 3.7)

1. The iliopectineal line
2. The ilioischial line
3. The teardrop (The medial portion of the teardrop represents the quadrilateral surface and the lateral portion represents the medial aspect of the acetabular floor)
4. The dome
5. The anterior wall
6. The posterior wall

Other Views: This includes the following views

- The obturator oblique radiograph (to view the anterior column and posterior wall) (Fig. 3.8)
- Iliac oblique radiograph (the posterior column and the anterior wall) (Fig. 3.9)
- Inlet view allows the surgeon to view anteroposterior displacement of the hemipelvis.
- The outlet view allows evaluation of superior and inferior displacement of the hemipelvis.

CT Scan

Two- and three-dimensional CT scans are useful in evaluating intraarticular fragments as well as specific morphologic characteristics of any given fracture pattern.

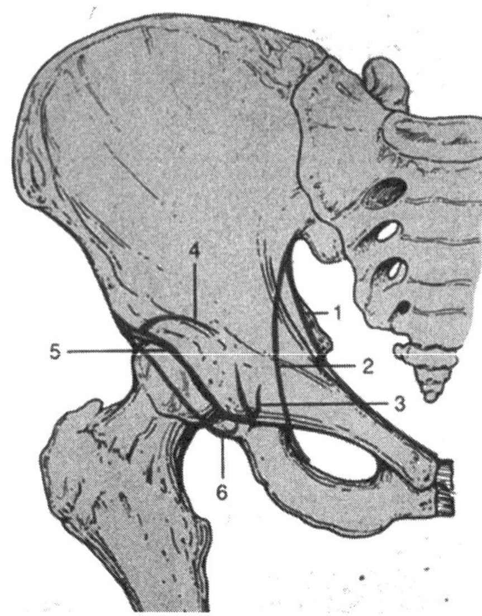

Fig. 3.7: The 6 major lines to be considered on the AP view of the pelvis (see page 31 for detail)

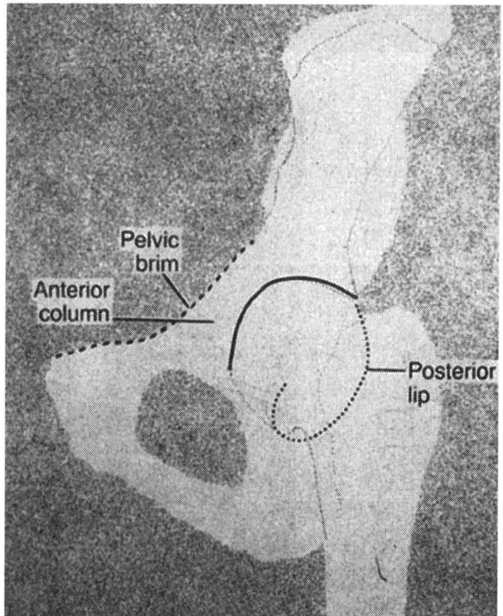

Fig. 3.8: Landmarks on the obturator oblique view

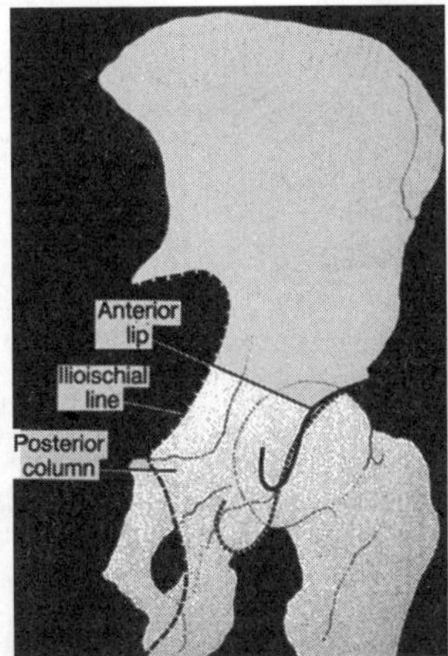

Fig. 3.9: Landmarks on the iliac oblique view

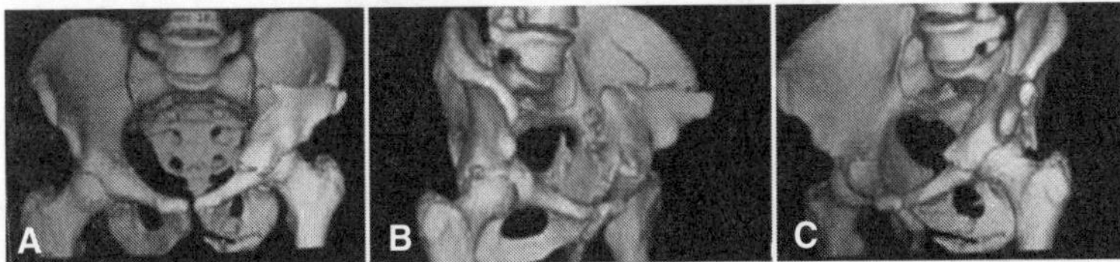

Figs 3.10A to C: CT Scan of the pelvis showing the acetabular fractures: (A) Anteroposterior view, (B) The iliac view, (c) The obturator view

Note: Posterior wall and posterior column fractures can be distinguished easily. In a posterior column fracture, the ilioischial line is interrupted, while only the retroacetabular surface is disrupted in a posterior wall fracture (Figs 3.11 and 3.12).

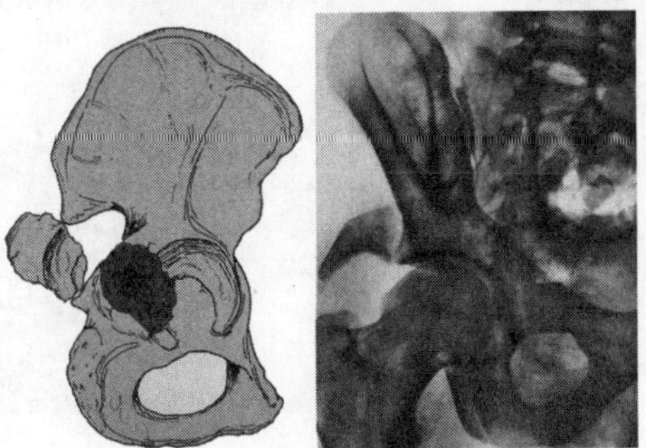

Fig. 3.11: Posterior wall fracture

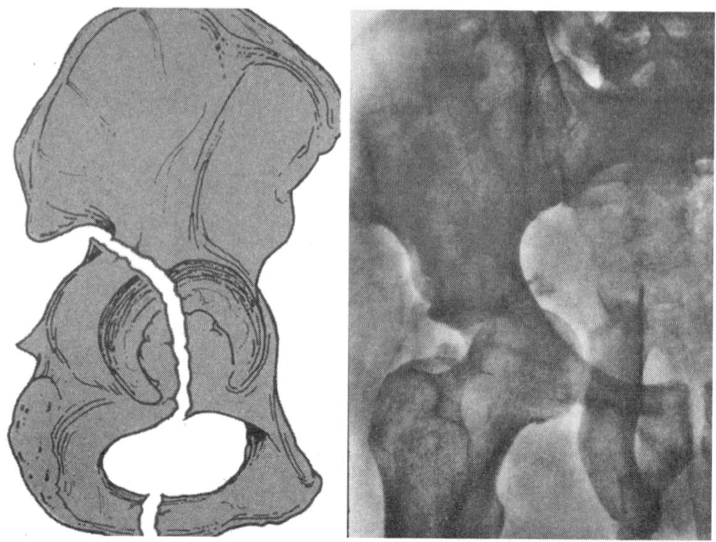

Fig. 3.12: Posterior wall fracture

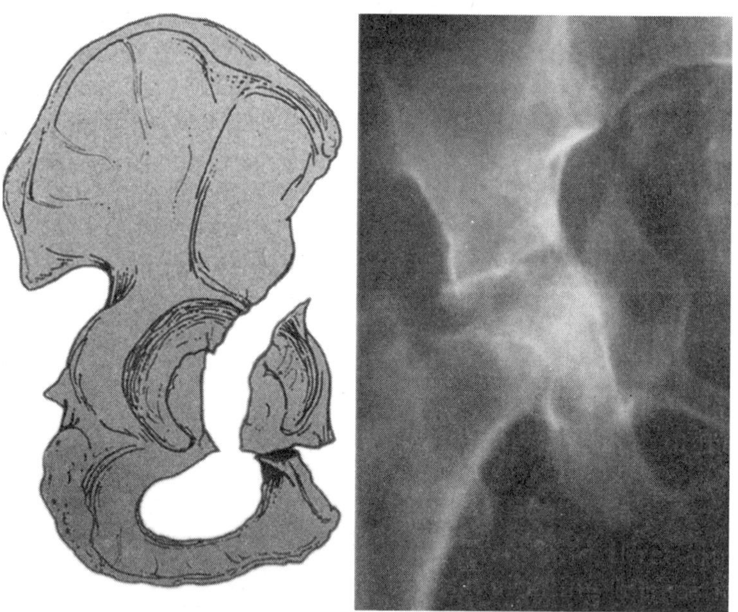

Fig. 3.13: Anterior wall fracture

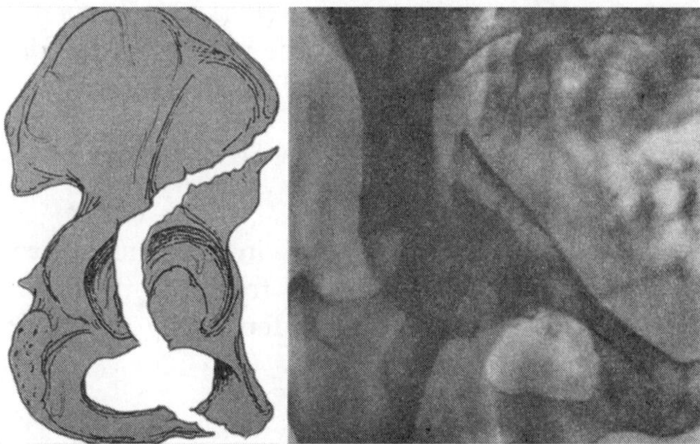

Fig. 3.14: Anterior column fracture

TRANSVERSE FRACTURES

A transverse acetabular fracture involves a fracture line that goes through both columns of the acetabulum, but a portion of the dome of the acetabulum remains attached to the constant fragment of the iliac wing (Fig. 3.15).

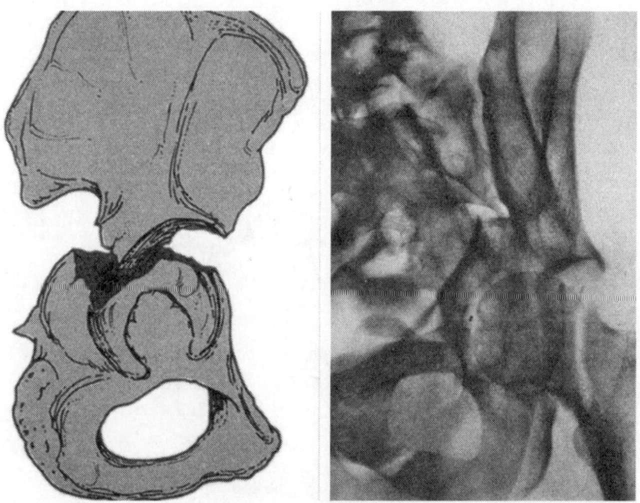

Fig. 3.15: Transverse fracture

Transverse acetabular fractures (Fig. 3.16): (depending on the orientation of the fracture line relative to the dome or tectum of the acetabulum) can be divided into

- Infratectal fractures (A)
- Juxtatectal (B)
- Transtectal (C)

Transtectal fractures are less forgiving and must be reduced anatomically, whereas infratectal fractures, if low enough, can be treated without surgery, depending on the pattern. (Fig. 3.16A to C)

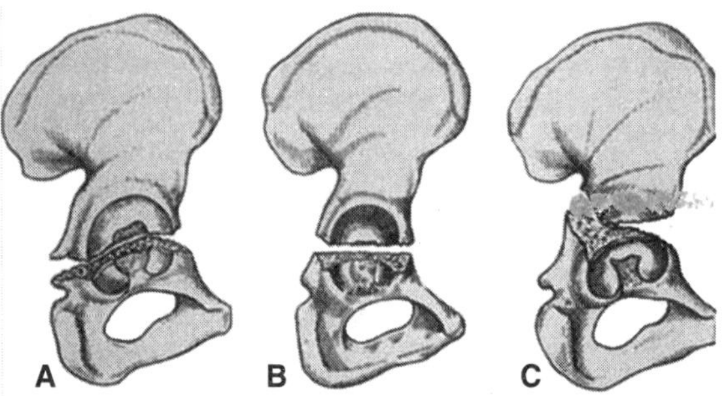

Figs 3.16A to C: Different types of transverse fracture

Note: Transverse fractures are sagittal plane fractures whereas both column fractures are coronal plane fractures (Figs 3.17 and 3.18)

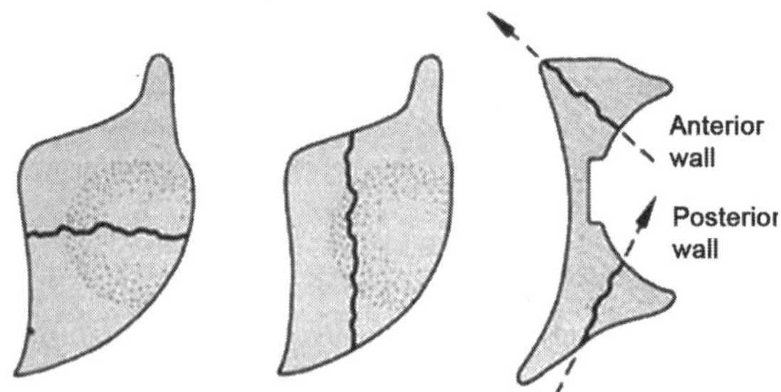

Fig. 3.17: Coronal plane fracture and sagittal plane fracture

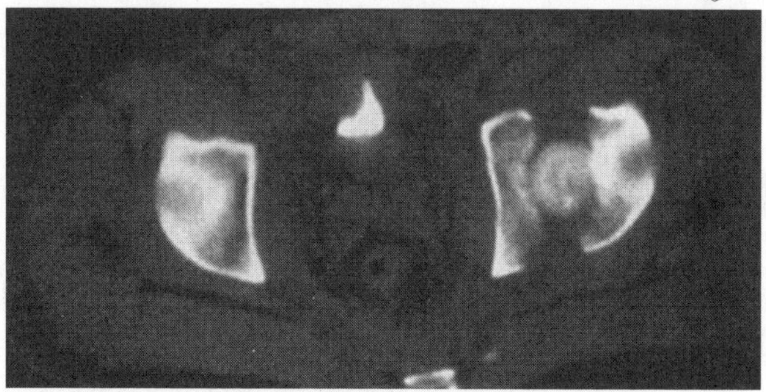

Fig. 3.18: CT cut of transverse fracture in the sagittal plane

T-TYPE FRACTURES

T-type fractures differ from transverse fractures by the additional fracture line that runs through the quadrilateral surface. As a result, the anterior column and posterior column are separated by fracture lines (Figs 3.19 and 3.20). In a T-type fracture, the 2 columns must be reduced independently.

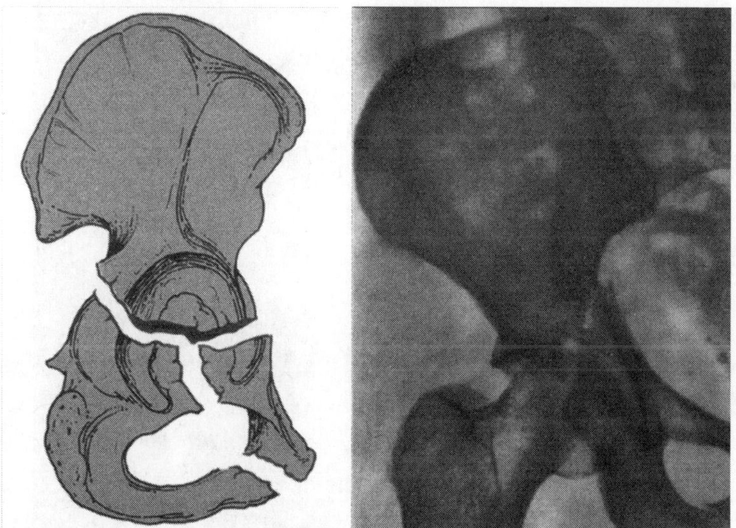

Fig. 3.19: T-type fracture

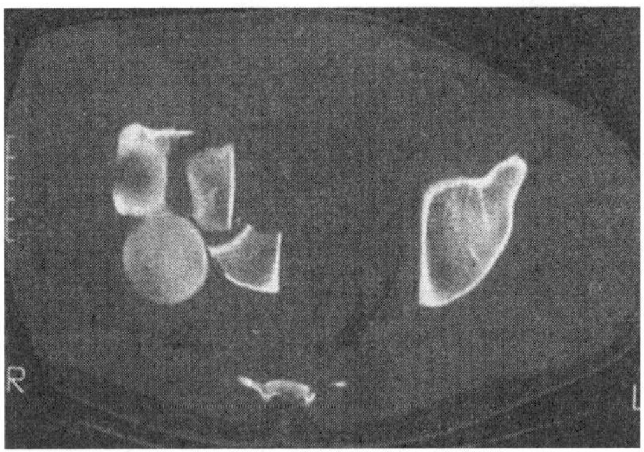

Fig. 3.20: 2-D CT cut of T-type fracture

Both-column Fractures

In a both-column fracture, the entire acetabulum is separated from the iliac wing. This is considered a "floating" acetabulum, and the "spur-sign," which is best seen on the obturator oblique view, is pathognomonic for the both-column fracture (Fig. 3.21).

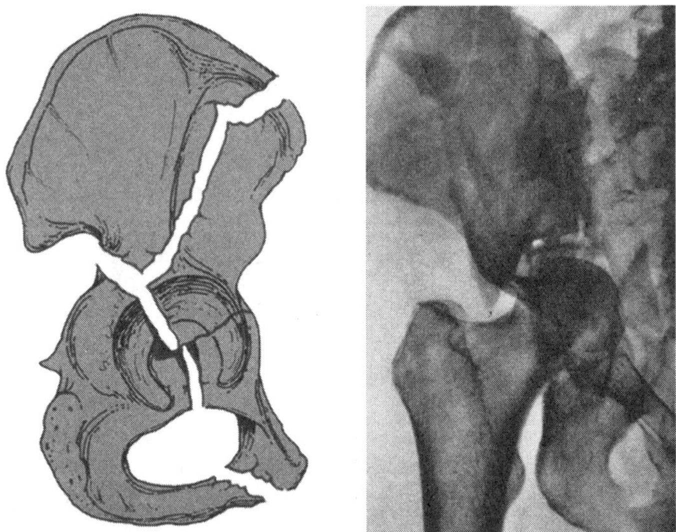

Fig. 3.21: Both-column fracture

AP, obturator oblique, and iliac oblique views showing a both-column acetabular fracture. The obturator oblique view shows the pathognomonic "spur-sign."

> *Note:* The spur represents the iliac wing fragment, or the constant fragment, and the entire acetabulum has been medialized. None of the dome of the acetabulum remains attached to the iliac wing.

Clinical Features

Vital parameters: Patient with acetabular fractures can present with injuries to the chest, abdomen, and cranium first because many acetabular fractures are associated with severe trauma.

Clinical Presentation

Symptoms: The patient may present with features of shock due to injuries to the vital organs as mentioned above and may complain of pain, swelling, deformity, inability to move, loss of movements of the affected hip joint, etc.

Clinical Signs

Attitude of the lower limb

- It is adducted, flexed, and internally rotated in a posterior dislocation.
- It is abducted and externally rotated in an anterior dislocation.
- Eversion of the iliac wing, with the anterior superior iliac spine on the affected side being more laterally placed, is a subtle clue to a central dislocation.

Skin may show local wounds, abrasions, and closed degloving injury.

Morel-Lavele lesion: This is a closed degloving injury occurring over the greater trochanter, in which the subcutaneous tissue is torn from underlying fascia creating a cavity, which places this tissue at risk for infection and/or poor healing.

Abduction and adduction of the hip: To detect instability manual traction can aid in determination of vertical instability.

Limb-length inequality: This may indicate the presence of incarcerated intra-articular fragments.

Neurologic examination: Needs to be done to exclude preoperative sciatic/lateral popliteal nerve palsy

Associated injuries: Associated injuries are also important to assess. Patients often have multiple traumatic injuries, and a high likelihood of associated injury exists in up to 50% of patients. One must diligently look for these injuries, as some are subtle and can be missed. Associated limb injuries could be

- Patella fracture
- Upper tibial fracture
- Posterior cruciate ligament injury.
- Associated femoral shaft fractures.
- Associated concomitant pelvic fractures may be present in up to 20% of patients.

Other injuries: It is also important to exclude injury to

- The bowel
- The urinary tract.

Treatment

I. Non-operative treatment should be considered in the following circumstances:

1. Undisplaced fractures.
2. Displaced fractures in the following situations:
   - A large portion of the acetabulum remains intact and the femoral head remains congruous with this portion of the acetabulum.

- A secondary congruence is present only after moderate displacement of a both-column fracture and the patient presents late (>3 week after injury).
- Small posterosuperior wall fractures that are associated with a stable hip joint and a congruent reduction. (Careful follow-up is needed to monitor for signs and symptoms of late instability in the initial months after injury.).
- A posterior wall injury that is minimally displaced or nondisplaced and is part of a more complex pattern requiring an ilioinguinal approach.
- If surgery is contraindicated (*see* contraindications).

II. Surgery

Indications for open reduction and internal fixation include the following:

- All displaced fractures (>2 mm articular step).
- Intact roof-arc angle less than 30°.
- Failure to achieve or maintain concentric reduction by closed means.
- Fractures that have a medial roof-arc angle of 45° or less, an anterior roof-arc angle of 25° or less, or a posterior roof-arc angle of 70° or less across the weight-bearing portion of the acetabulum, according to Vrahas et al, on the basis of a cadaveric study; persistent instability after closed reduction.
- Incarcerated intra-articular fragments or impaction of the articular surface.
- Emergency open reduction and internal fixation (ORIF) if associated vascular injury or sciatic palsy develops after a closed reduction.

Contraindications: Surgery include the following:

- General: Severe systemic illness or secondary multiorgan failure secondary to polytrauma; systemic infections or sepsis
- Local: Local infection; extreme osteoporosis.

- Relative: Severe comminution; pre-existing arthrosis

Surgical intervention may be carried out in these cases to facilitate a salvage procedure later.

Surgical Approaches

For anterior column fractures: The ileo-inguinal or the ileo-femoral approaches.

For posterior column fractures: The Kellegreen-Lewis approach is used for fixing the posterior column fractures. (Fig. 3.22).

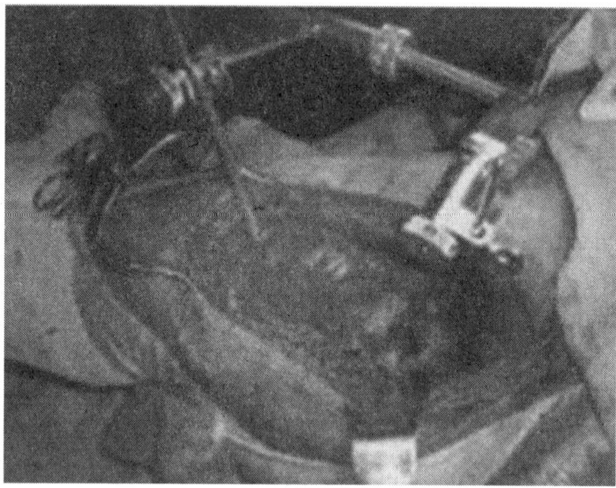

Fig. 3.22: The posterior KL approach for fixation of posterior column fractures

The implants used for fixation are the reconstruction plates, semitubular plates and cortical screws (Fig. 3.23).

Complications

Immediate complications include shock, fat embolism, injuries to the vital organs, death, etc. Delayed complications include secondary OA of the hip, etc.

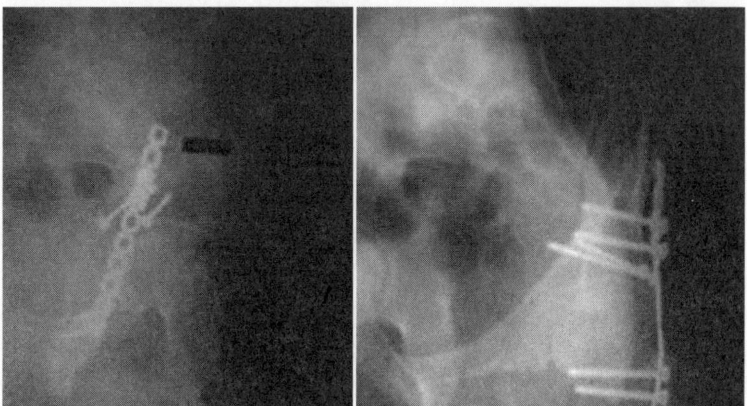

Fig. 3.23: Fixation of anterior and posterior column acetabular fractures with reconstruction plate and screws

4 Injuries Around the Hip Joint

Dislocations and Fracture Dislocations

Introduction

When God designed the 65 joints in a human body, he made the hip joint very big and strong to support the weight on a biped stance. Consequently considerable force is required to bring it out of its socket. These forces are provided 70–100 percent of the times by high-speed motor vehicle accidents. Though hip dislocations were reported earlier to the discovery of the X-rays, it was Funsten in 1938 that first reported a series of 20 hip dislocations and also coined the term "dashboard dislocation". In his series and in subsequent series by other authors, it was found that these dislocations usually happen when the knees of the front seat occupants in a vehicle strike against the dashboard of the vehicle usually in a head on collision. Depending on the position of the limb at the time of impact, there could be either pure dislocation or fracture dislocation. The enormity of the trauma could also cause multisystem injuries of the head, trunk, abdomen, pelvis, etc.

Look what could happen in hip dislocations?

- Pure hip dislocations.
- Fracture hip dislocations: Fracture acetabulum, fracture head of femur, fracture neck of femur.
- *Other injuries:* Knee ligament injuries, fracture patella, supracondylar fracture femur, shaft femur, etc.
- Other limb fractures.
- Multisystem injuries.
- Pelvic fractures, rib fractures, spine fractures, etc.

Now you know why managing hip dislocations is a gigantic challenge to a treating orthopedic surgeon. Depending upon the presentation it may be a solo or a multimodality and multispecialty approach. Nonetheless hip dislocations are an emergency amidst life threatening emergencies if any and needs to be treated on a top priority basis. If hip joint is 'out' pushing it back 'in' should be the mantra lest troublesome delayed complications like AVN, degenerative arthritis, etc. stare in your face.

CLINICAL SIGNIFICANCE OF VASCULAR ANATOMY

Avascular necrosis of femoral head and post-traumatic degenerative hip are the two very important and common complications of hip dislocations. A thorough knowledge of the vascular anatomy is a must to understand the reasons behind (Fig. 4.1). Femoral head circulation is through three sources:

- Intraosseous cervical vessels.

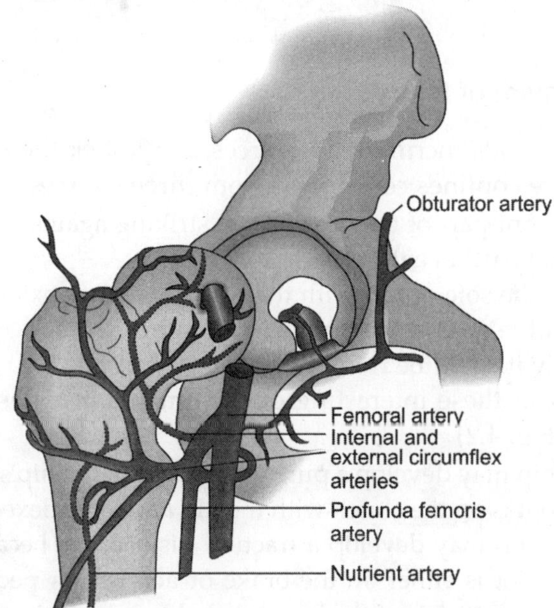

Fig. 4.1: Vascular anatomy of the hip joint (From Paul Levin, MD)

- Artery of ligamentum teres.
- Retinacular vessels (Man supply).

If there is damage to these vessels during dislocation, or during reduction and also due to the delay in diagnosis and treatment, this could lead to avascular necrosis of the femoral head and later to degenerative arthritis.

"Therefore, the aim of treatment is early anatomical reduction to protect the existing circulation of the head of the femur."

Causes

- High speed RTA's.
- Violent falls from heights.
- Sports related injuries.
- Industrial accidents.
- Natural calamities, etc.

Note: Nearly 70–100 percent of the hip dislocations are due to RTA.

Mechanism of Injury

The notorious incriminating forces that knock the hips out of its safe confines could arise from three sources:

- The front part of the flexed knee striking against an object (dash board events).
- From the sole of feet with the ipsilateral knee extended.
- From the greater trochanter.
- Rarely it could be from the posterior pelvis.

Look at these interesting developments in a dashboard injury (Fig. 4.2)

- Left hip may develop a pure dislocation of the hip since the left foot is on the clutch with the hip and knee flexed at 90°.
- Right hip may develop a fracture dislocation, because the right foot is either on the brake or accelerator pedal with the hip in 60–70° of flexion and slight abduction.

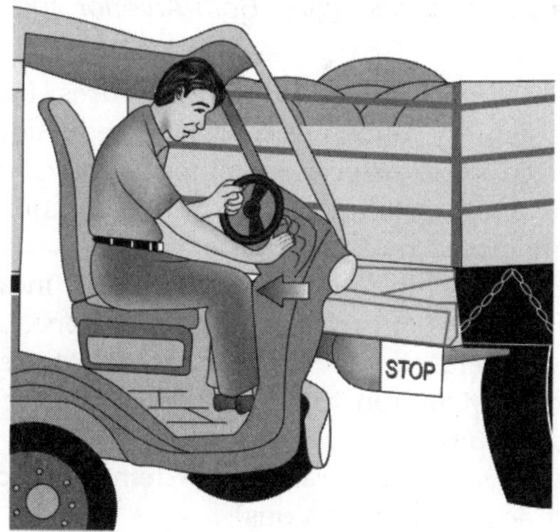

Fig. 4.2: The dashboard injury

Classification

Depending upon the position of the head with respect to the acetabulum, hip dislocations are classified as

- *Posterior dislocations:* Commonest and is seen in 80–90 percent of the cases.
- *Anterior dislocations:* Seen in 10–15 percent.
- *Central dislocations:* Relatively rare.

Overall Classification of the Hip Dislocations (Stewart and Milfort, based on the hip stability and femoral head condition, both anterior and posterior)

Type I: Dislocates with either no fracture or an insignificant ace tabular rim fracture.

Type II: Dislocations with either a single or a communized posterior wall fracture but the hip is stable.

Type III: Fracture dislocations with gross instability due to loss of structural support.

Type IV: Dislocations with femoral head fracture.

Comprehensive Classification—Both Anterior and Posterior (Fig. 4.3)

Type I: No significant associated fractures, no clinical instability following concentric reduction.

Type II: Irreducible dislocation without significant femoral hear or acetabular fracture (reduction must be attempted under GA).

Type III: Unstable hip following reduction or incarcerated fragments of cartilage, labrum or bone.

Type IV: Associated acetabular fracture requiring reconstruction to restore hip stability or joint congruity.

Type V: Associated femoral hear or femoral neck injury (fracture or impactions).

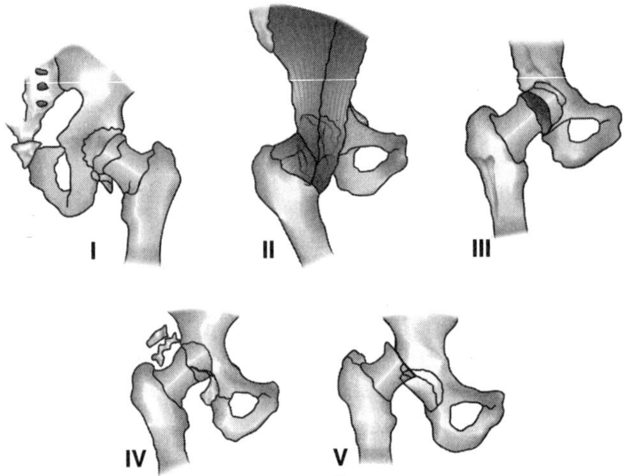

Figs 4.3: The comprehensive classification of posterior dislocation of the hip (Types I to V) (From Paul Levin, MD)

POSTERIOR HIP DISLOCATIONS

As mentioned earlier this is the most common variety of hip dislocations. The dislocation could be simple or may be associated with fracture dislocations.

Thompson and Epstein have further classified the posterior dislocation of the hip into four types and Pipkin has given four sub-classifications for the femoral head fracture in type IVB fracture of the Thompson and Epstein variety.

THOMPSON AND EPSTEIN CLASSIFICATIONS

(Fig. 4.4)

Type I: With or without minor fracture.

Type II: With a large single fracture of the posterior acetabular rim.

Type III: With comminution of the rim of the acetabulum with or without a major fragment.

Type IV: With fracture of the acetabular floor.

Type V: With fracture of the femoral head. This has been further classified by Pipkin into four types.

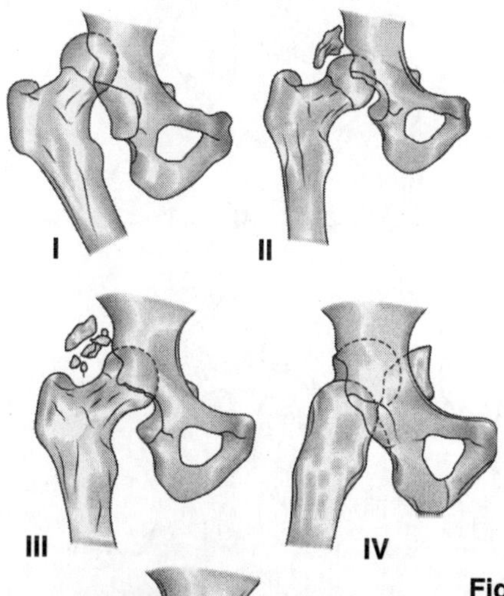

Fig. 4.4: Thompson and Epstein's classification of posterior hip dislocations (Types I to V) (From Delee, J.C. Fractures and dislocations. In: Rockwood, CA, Jr: Green, DP Fractures, Vol. 2, 2nd ed, JB Lippincott, 1985)

PIPKIN TYPES (Dislocation of the hip with fractures of the femoral head) (Fig. 4.5)

Type I: Femoral dislocation of the hip with fracture of the femoral head caudad to the fovea centralis.

Type II: Posterior dislocation of the hip with fracture of the femoral head cephalad to the fovea centralis.

Type III: Type I and Type II with associated fracture of the femoral neck.

Type IV: Types I, II or III with associated facture of the acetabulum.

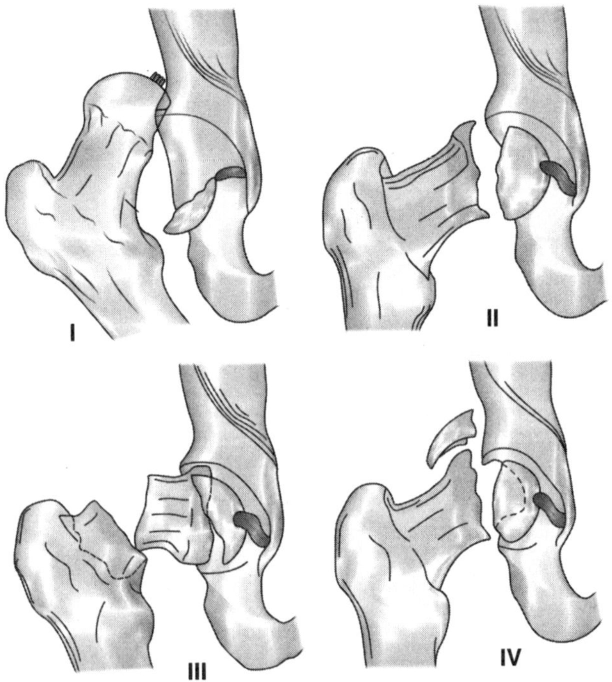

Fig. 4.5: Types I to IV Pipkin's classification (From Delee, JC Fractures and dislocations. In: Rockwood, CA, Jr: Green, DP Fractures, Vol. 2, 2nd ed, JB Lippincott, 1985)

Clinical Features

There is usually history of trauma and the patient has a flexion, adduction and medial rotation deformity of the affected limb (Figs 4.6A and B). There is marked shortening and gross restriction of all hip movements. Head of the femur is felt as a hard mass in the gluteal region and it moves along with the femur. There could be features of sciatic nerve palsy. It may be difficult to feel the femoral pulse (Vascular sign of Narath is negative). In fracture posterior hip dislocation, this classical presentation may not be seen.

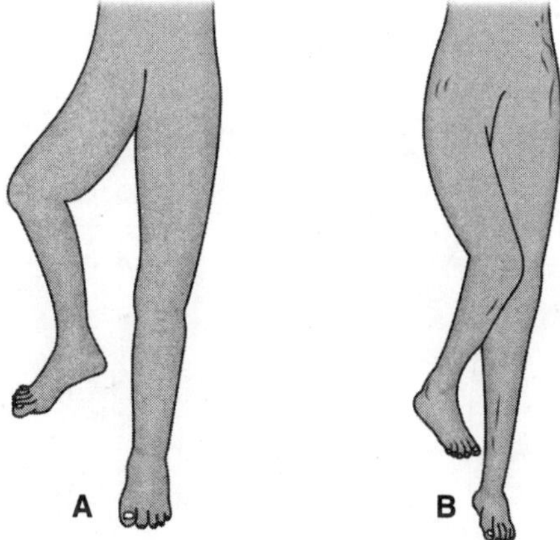

Figs 4.6A and B: Appearance of classical deformities in dislocation hip: (A) Anterior, and (B) Posterior

Investigations

Before Reduction

Laboratory tests: Hb percent, BT, CT, Blood group, RBS, etc. needs to be done as for any other major surgery.

Plain X-ray of the hip: All high-energy trauma and multiple injury patients should have a screening AP view of the pelvis.

What to look for in the initial X-ray:
- Are the femoral heads symmetric in size?
- Is the joint space symmetric throughout?
- Is the head large (anterior dislocation) or small (posterior dislocation)?
- Is the Shenton' line maintained or broken? (Fig. 4.7)
- Is the greater trochanter prominent (posterior) or inconspicuous (anterior) reverse with lesser trochanter?
- Is the femoral neck normal?

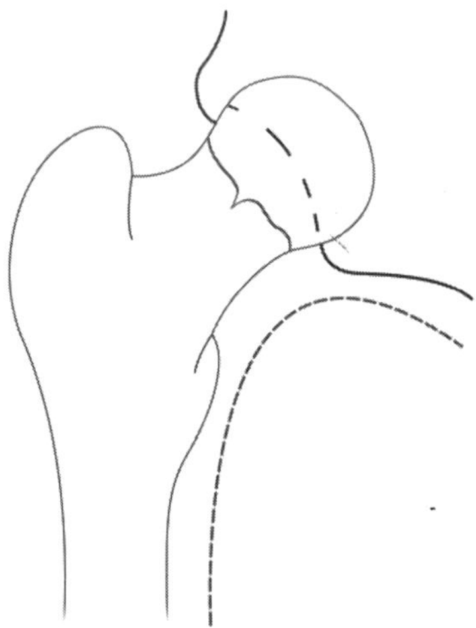

Fig. 4.7: Shenton's line

After Reduction

Plain X-ray of the hip
- AP X-ray centered on the affected hip (Fig. 4.8).
- Judet views with the affected hip in internal and external oblique views at 45 degrees.

What to look for?
- Is there any incarcerated osteochondral fragment within the joint?

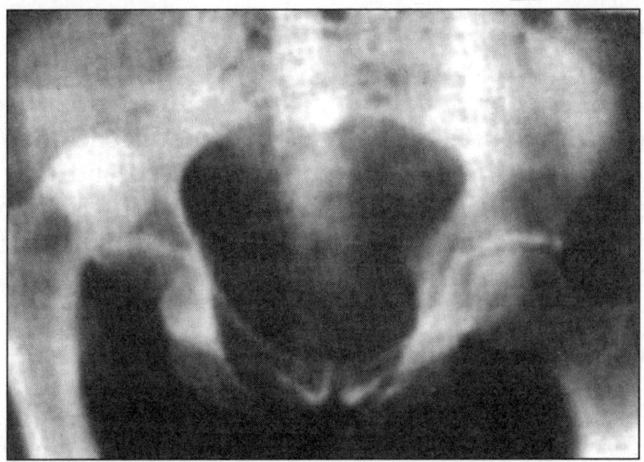

Fig. 4.8: Radiograph showing posterior dislocation of the hip joint

- Is the joint space asymmetric?
- Look for the anterior and posterior ace tabular wall.
- Look for any indentation on the femoral head.

CT scan: CT Scan should be routinely done after a successful or failed closed reduction. The importance of CT lies in:
- Assessing the femoral head.
- To demonstrate the presence of small intra-articular fragments.
- To assess the congruence of the femoral head and acetabulum.
- Osteochondral fractures, occult impactions, indentations and other fractures are easily seen on a CT.

MRI: This has its limitations in the acute evaluation of the multiple injured patients. However, as an adjunct to CT, it helps to evaluate the integrity of the labrum and assess the vascularity of the femoral head.

Bone scan: This has a limited and questionable role in hip dislocations.

Management

All hip dislocations are emergencies and need to be reduced within 6–12 hours following injury to prevent troublesome late complications like AVN and traumatic degenerative hip. Once reduction is done urgency is reduced and now the diagnostic workup, CT scan and surgical intervention if necessary can all be done once the general condition of the patient is stabilized.

Goal of Treatment

Prompt reduction of the femoral head.

Types of reduction: This is either closed or open. Thompson-Epstein believed that closed reduction should be reserved for simple hip dislocations and open reduction for hip dislocations, while majority of the authors believe that closed reduction should be tried initially in all cases of simple and fracture dislocation and open reduction shoulder be reserved for the patients in whom;

- Closed reduction fails.
- Reduction is unstable.
- After reduction, if there are trapped fracture fragments within the joint.

Type I Dislocation

Here prompt closed reduction of the hip is the treatment of choice.

Methods of Closed Reduction

There are various techniques described in the literature. The important methods are the ABCS.

A – Allis method
B – Bigelow method
C – Classical Watson-Jones method
S – Stimson's gravity method

Note: All the reductions should be done under General Anesthesia.

Now let us try to know each method of reduction in greater detail.

A. Allis Method (Fig. 4.9)

- Patient is supine.
- An assistant stabilizes the pelvis by applying pressure on both the ASIS.
- Traction is applied in the line of the deformity.
- The hip is gently flexed to 90 degrees.
- The hip is now gently rotated, internally and externally, with continued longitudinal traction till reduction is achieved.

Bass's Method (Modified Allis method): This is the flexion adduction method. With the patient under general anesthesia, the hip is flexed to 90 degrees in maximum adduction as the longitudinal traction is applied in the axis of the femur while an assistant stabilizes the pelvis.

B. Bigelow's Method (Fig. 4.10)

- Patient is supine.
- An assistant applies counter traction on both the ASIS.

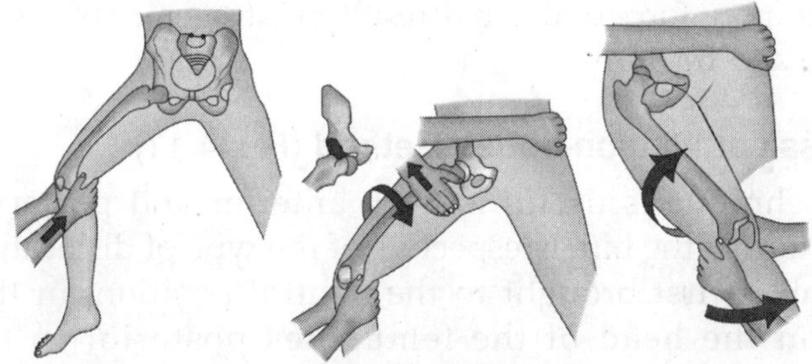

Fig. 4.9: Technique of Allis method of reduction of the hip dislocation (From Delee, JC Fractures and Dislocations. In: Rockwood, CA, Jr: Green, DP Fractures, Vol.2, 2nd ed, JB Lippincott, 1985)

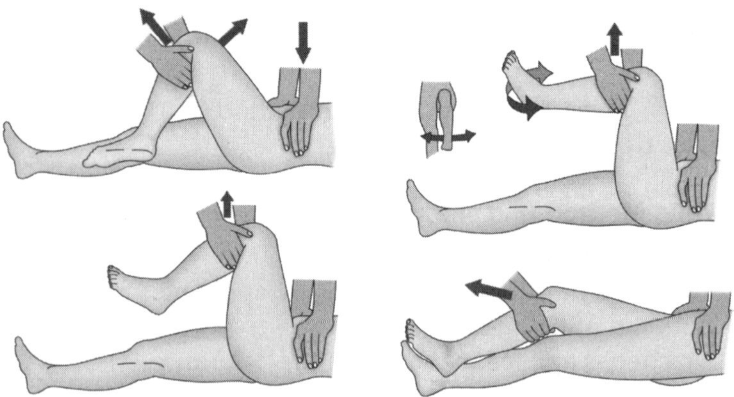

Fig. 4.10: Bigelow's method of reduction (From Delee, JC Fractures In adults: Eds Rockwood and Green, 1996)

- Surgeon applies longitudinal traction in the line of the deformity.
- The hip is gently adducted, internally rotated and bent on the abdomen. This relaxes the Y-ligament and brings the femoral head near the poster inferior aspect of the acetabulum.
- By adduction, external rotation and extension of the hip, head is levered back into the acetabulum.

Caution: This technique should be done with lot of care, as it requires more force and could result in iatrogenic soft tissue damage and fractures.

C. Classical Watson-Jones Method (Fig. 4.11)

This technique is useful in both anterior and posterior dislocation of the hip. Irrespective of the type of dislocation the limb is first brought to the neutral position. In this position the head of the femur lies posterior to the acetabulum even in anterior dislocation. Now with an assistant steadying the pelvis the head of the femur is reduced into the acetabulum by applying a longitudinal traction in the long axis of the femur. It is simple and effective when compared to Bigelow's method.

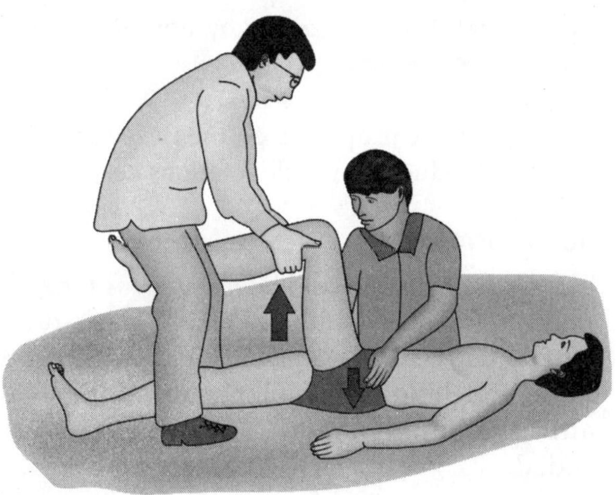

Fig. 4.11: Watson-Jones classical method of reduction

D. Stimson's Gravity Method (Fig. 4.12)

In reality this is the reverse Allis method of reduction. The steps are as follows:

- Patient is prone.
- Patient is brought to the edge of the table.

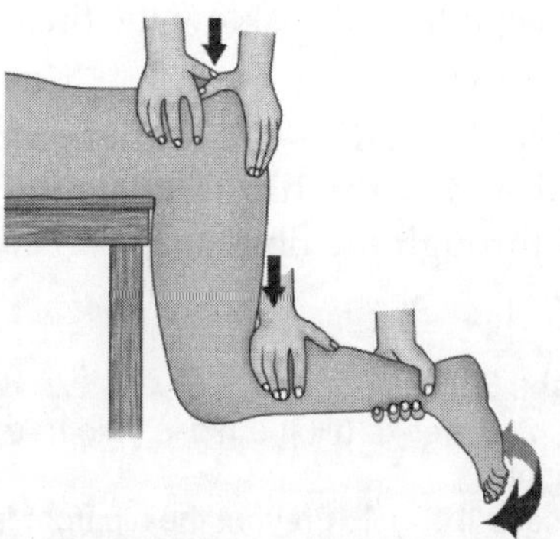

Fig. 4.12: Stimson's gravity method of reduction (From Delee, JC Fractures and dislocations. In: Rockwood, CA, Jr: Green, DP Fractures, Vol.2, 2nd ed, JB Lippincott, 1985)

- An assistant stabilizes the pelvis by applying downward pressure over the sacrum.
- The affected hip and knees are flexed to 90 degrees.
- Downward pressure is applied on the flexed knee.
- To facilitate the reduction, gentle rotations needs to be done.

Postreduction Protocol

Radiographic verifications: AP and lateral views of the affected hip and pelvis AP views should be taken. The X-ray has to be carefully evaluated for the concentric reduction by looking for the subtle widening of the joint space. If there are any significant acetabular factures, Judet views are recommended.

Evaluation of the postreduction stability: After the radiographic verification of the dislocation, a stability check is carried out as follows:

- Flex the hip to 90–95 degrees in neutral, abduction and adduction and rotation.
- A strong posterior force is thus applied.
- If there is evidence of subluxation, additional diagnostic studies are required and surgical exploration or traction may be required at a later date.

Postreduction CT evaluation: This is very important and the role of CT has already been discussed. Now the final staging of the hip dislocation is carried out.

Postreduction traction: If the hip is stable after reduction, Buck's traction is applied and if the hip is unstable then skeletal traction is applied through the tibia pin.

Traction facts

- Permissible weight: 5 to 8 pounds.
- Permissible time: 2–3 weeks (till the hip is pain free and has good range of movements).
- Traction requirement: It should prevent the hip from flexion, internal rotation and adduction.
- Weight bearing can be resumed after 2–4 weeks once the pain and spasm disappears.

Bad news for spica cast: Spica cast should not be used for postreduction stabilization. Since it prevents early range of movements necessary to promote healing. This damages the articular cartilage and leads to post-traumatic arthritis in future.

Treatment of Type II, III and IV: Here there is an argument over the closed vs. open reduction. Most authors' worldwide feel that hip dislocations with acetabular fractures should be reduced at the earliest. This they claim gives a better long-term outcome than operative reduction. However, Epstein recommends early primary open reduction and he claims better results with this approach. However, theoretically acceptable, practically it has its lacunae as optimum operating conditions for major hip procedure as an emergency procedure is seldom found. If open reduction is warranted it can always be done later, after stabilizing the patient without compromising on the longterm safety of the patients.

Whether the choice is closed or open reduction techniques for posterior fracture dislocations, the following factors are prognostically important

- Degree of initial trauma.
- Reduction either closed or open should be performed within 12–24 hours.
- If closed reduction is the choice, it has to be attempted only once failing which open reduction should be attempted.

Indications for Open Reduction

- Failed closed reduction.
- Failed stability test.
- Big posterior lip fragment.
- Bone fragment within the acetabulum.
- Fracture of the femoral head.
- Sciatic nerve palsy.

Technique of Open Reduction

- Approach: Posterior approach is favored though some have tried anterior Watson-Jones or transtrochanteric approach.

- Debridement: Joint is thoroughly irrigated to remove all pieces of bone and cartilage.
- Reduction of the hip, if it has not been done previously.
- Reposition of the fracture fragments carefully and reconstruct the acetabulum.
- In Type II injury with the large Acetabular chunk can be fixed by a single cancellous screws.
- In Type III with several pieces reconstruction is attempted as accurately as possible and fixation is done with cancellous screws or small malleable plate, etc.
- In severe comminution reconstruction is done through a full thickness iliac graft/autograft.
- In type IV fractures are fixed based on the location and Epstein claims poor results in these cases irrespective of the type of treatment.

Postoperative Treatment

- Skeletal traction (10–15 lb) with the hip in slight abduction and extension.
- Within 3–5 days, gentle active and passive exercises in traction are begun.
- Traction to be maintained for 6–8 weeks.
- Later protected weight bearing is allowed.

Type V Posterior Fracture Dislocations

- There is associated femoral head fracture.
- First reported by Birkett in 1869.
- Incidence is 6–7 percent.
- Incidence is on the rise due to increase in RTA's.

Mechanism of Injury

- In a dashboard injury if the hip is in 60 degrees of flexion or less and is in neutral position it could result in a combined dislocation and fracture of the femoral head.
- Avulsion of the femoral head through an intact ligamentum teres.

Classification

Pipkin's types: Here posterior dislocation of hip could be associated with fracture head of the femur and has been discussed earlier.

Management

Type I

- Closed reduction is often successful. Pipkin has suggested after closed reduction the fragments return back to their normal anatomical position.
- Surgical excision if the displaced femoral head fracture obstructs the reduction Pipkin noted that degenerative changes in the caudal fragment have no bearing in the long-term result.

Type II: According to Swintkwoski in Pipkin I and II, if the displacement of the fracture is less than 2 mm on postreduction CT scan.

Methods of Treatment

- Primary closed reduction.
- Excision (Epstein): If the fragment is less than one-third of the articular surface.
- Open reduction and internal fixation in large fragments. This is indicated if the femoral head fracture cannot be reduced by closed means. Internal fixation is done by Herbert Screws.

In this injury since the ligamentum teres is still attached to the head fragment, blood supply to the fragment is still maintained and it heals well.

Type III: Only 13 cases have been reported in the literature and 5 of these were iatrogenic and happened at the time of performing the closed reduction for the hip dislocation. These fractures can be treated as follows:

- Open reduction and internal fixation of the femoral neck fracture. The femoral head fractures were then treated as in Types I and II.

- These can also be treated as primary insertion of endoprosthesis or other types of arthroplasty.

Type IV: Here there is associated fracture of the acetabulum and fracture of the femoral head could be Type I/II/III. The treatment plan is dictated by the degree of ace tabular cartilage damage. Small fragments can be excised and the larger fragment needs to be fixed with screws. Later femoral head fracture is treated as in I and II.

Complications

Myositis ossificans (2%): It is seen commonly in posterior dislocation with head injury and is unknown in simple posterior dislocation. It may be seen after reduction also. It can be prevented by avoiding repeated manipulation, early immobilization and by immobilizing for 6 weeks in hip spica.

Sciatic nerve injury: Incidence of this injury is 10 to 13 percent (Fig. 4.13). It is 3 times more common in fracture dislocation than simple dislocation. Usually, it is a neuropraxia and the peroneal division is commonly affected. It may be due to stretch of the nerve or may be due to impalement between the fracture fragments. If it is associated with acetabular fracture the nerve should be explored. Prognosis is variable.

Traumatic osteoarthritis due to avascular necrosis (35%): For head of the femur major blood supply enters from the capsule and to a lesser extent through the ligamentum teres. If both these sources are damaged, it gradually leads to AVN followed by osteoarthritis of the hip joint. Incidence is about 10 percent.

Recurrent dislocation: This is due to fracture acetabulum and sometimes due to rent in the capsule and gluteus minimus. This requires exploration and fixing of the acetabular fragments with screws.

Unreduced dislocation: This is common in Asian patients due to ignorance and illiteracy. Manipulative reduction is tried first. If it is unsuccessful operative reduction is attempted. Arthrodesis if acceptable is the best treatment. Total hip

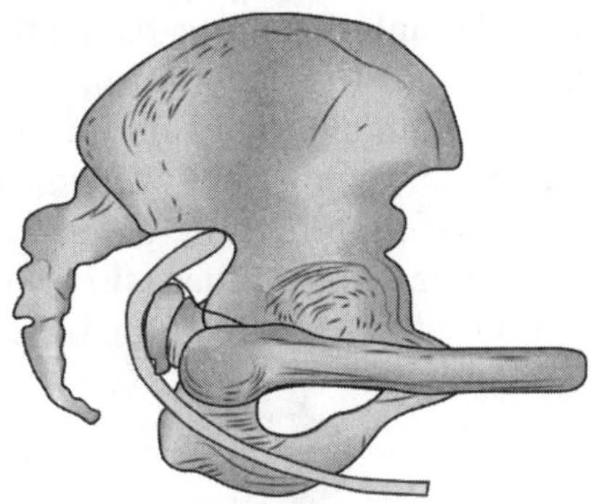

Fig. 4.13: Sciatic nerve injury in posterior dislocation of the hip

replacement is usually not preferred because the patient is usually young. In hips where there is useful range of painless movements corrective osteotomy is done. In painful stiff joints, girdlestone excision is preferred.

Irreducible dislocation (31%): This may be due to bony (acetabular fragments, femoral head, etc.) or soft tissue (acetabular labrum, etc.) obstruction. It may also be due to coma, ipsilateral fracture femur or dislocation of opposite hip. It may require exploration and open reduction.

ANTERIOR DISLOCATION OF THE HIP

Incidence: This is rare and is seen in 10–15 percent of the cases.

Causes

- In RTA's, when the knee strikes the dashboard with the thigh abducted.
- Violent fall from the height.
- Forceful blow to the back of the patient in a squatted position (Fig. 4.14).

Mechanism of Injury

Due to the above forces, the neck of femur or the greater trochanter impinges on the rim of the acetabulum and through a tear in the anterior hip capsule; the head of the femur is levered out of the acetabulum. If the hip is in simultaneous abduction, external rotation and flexion, an inferior type (obturator) of dislocation results. And on the contrary if the hip is in abduction, external rotation and extension, it results in a pubic or iliac (superior) dislocation. There could be associated fracture of the head of the femur.

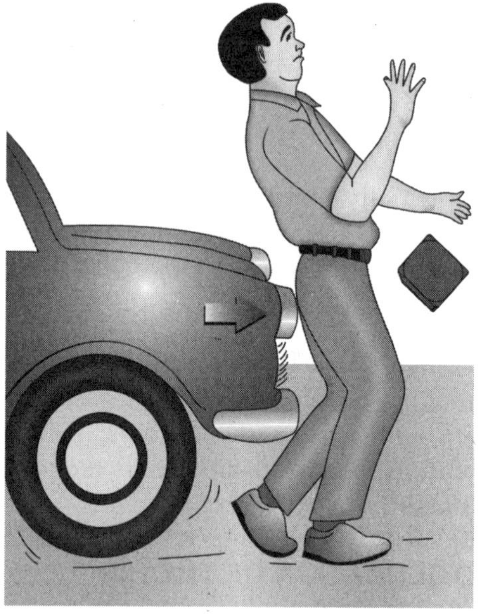

Fig. 4.14: Mechanism of injury in anterior dislocation of the hip

Classification

Comprehensive classification: This is same as for the posterior dislocation of the hip discussed earlier (Figs 4.15A to E) .

Epstein's Classification

Type I : Superior dislocation (includes pubic and subspinous dislocation).

Type IA : No associated fracture (Simple dislocation).

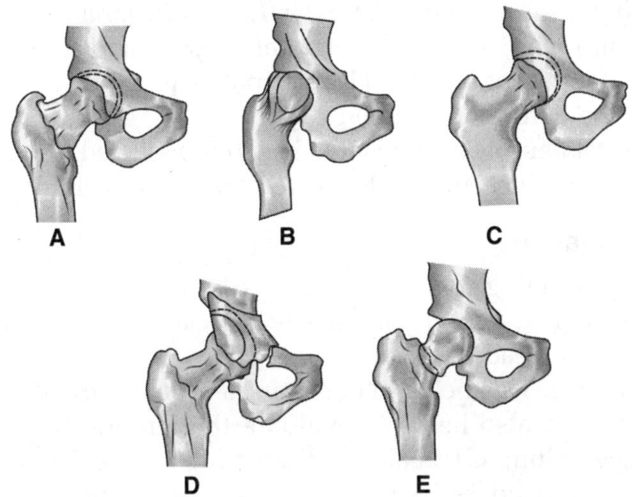

Figs 4.15A to E: Comprehensive classification of the anterior dislocation of the hip (From Paul Levin, MD)

Type IB : Associated facture of the head (transchondral or indentation type) and/or neck of the femur.

Type IC : Associated fracture of the acetabulum.

Type II : Inferior dislocation (includes obturator, thyroid and perineal dislocation).

Type IIA: No associated fracture (Simple dislocation).

Type IIB : Associated fracture of the head (transchondral or indentation type) and/or neck of the femur.

Type IIC: Associated fracture of the acetabulum.

Clinical Features

- Multisystem injuries is a possibility and has to be carefully evaluated.
- Position of the limb suggests the diagnosis
  - *In the superior type (Iliac or Pubic):* The hip is extended and externally rotated and the head is felt near the anterosuperior iliac spine in the iliac type and in the groin in the pubic type.

–In the inferior type (Obturator/Thyroid/Perineal): Here the hip is in abduction, external rotation and in varying degrees of flexion. Head is palpable in the region of the obturator foramen.

- Distal neurovascular status has to be assessed due to the possibility of injuries to the femoral vessels and nerve.

Investigations

- *X-ray:* Diagnosis can be easily made on a plain X-ray (Fig. 4.16). Look for any associated damage to the femoral head, neck, etc.
- *CT Scan:* This helps to detect intra-articular fragments if any and also helps to evaluate the femoral head and acetabulum. CT is also indicated after closed reduction or if closed reduction fails before doing the open reduction.
- *MRI:* This helps to evaluate the integrity of the labrum, vascularity of the femoral head and osteochondral lesion if any. It has a definite role in these cases of unstable hip after dislocation or in widened joint space after reduction.

Treatment

Goal: Prompt diagnosis and immediate closed reduction under general anesthesia.

Caution: Single and not multiple attempts are advised, failure warrants open reduction at the earliest.

Methods: ABCDS Method of Reduction

- *Allis method:* This is the same as for the posterior dislocation
- *Bigelow's method (Actually this is a reverse Bigelow):* Here the hip is in partial flexion and abduction. He has described two methods:
  - *The traction method:* Here the traction is applied in the line of the deformity and the hip is adducted, internally rotated and extended.

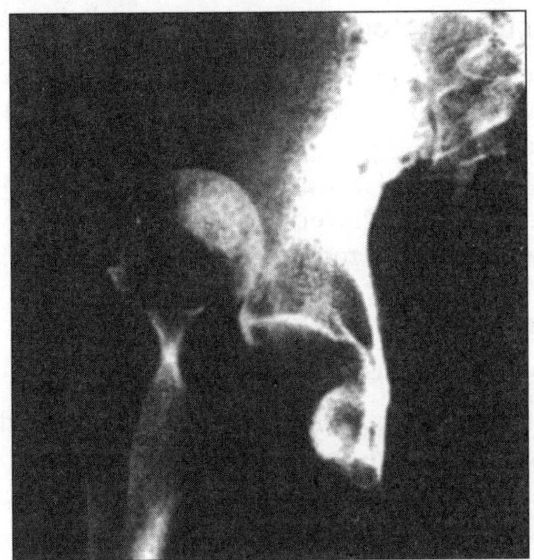

Fig. 4.16: Radiograph showing the iliac type of anterior dislocation of the hip

- *The lifting method:* Here a flexed thigh is lifted with a sudden jerk. However, this method is not successful in pubic dislocations.

- *Classical Watson-Jones' method:* This is the same as described previously in posterior dislocation of the hip.
- *Delee and Epstein method:* This is a modified Allis technique. It consists of continuous traction in the line of the deformity, hip in slight flexion, lateral force to the thigh with slight internal rotation and adduction.
- *Stimson's gravity method:* Same as for posterior dislocation. However, it is not useful in superior dislocation as the hip here is in an extended position. A careful X ray evaluation is must after closed reduction. Look for any associated transchondral fracture, femoral neck or head fracture. A transchondral fracture needs excision; open reduction an internal fixation for a large fracture of the femoral head and indentation fracture needs to be left alone.

Postreduction Protocol

- Traction for a period of 1–6 weeks.
- Controlled range of movements is instituted during the traction.
- Avoid extremes of abduction and external rotation.
- If there are associated fractures, longer period of immobilization are required.

Complications

Immediate complications: These are as follows:

Neurovascular compromise: In superior and open dislocations, there could be pressure on the femoral artery, vein and nerve leading to distal neurovascular compromise. It warrants immediate reduction of the hip dislocations.

Irreducibility: These could be due to the following reasons:
- Bony block in the obturator foramen.
- Soft tissue interposition could be from rectus femoris, iliopsoas muscle and anterior hip capsule. This necessitates open reduction.

Delayed Complications

Post-traumatic arthritis: This is reported in more than one-third to one-half of cases and the reasons could be:
- Femoral head fractures
- Acetabular fractures
- AVN
- Transchondral and indentation fractures.

AVN
- Incidence is 8 percent
- Less common than posterior dislocation
- May appear 2–5 years later
- Reasons could be due to delay or repeated attempts at reduction
- Extent of initial injury has an important role.

Recurrent dislocations: Defective capsular healing due to inadequate immobilization could lead to recurrent dislocations.

Unreduced dislocations: Commonly seen in developing condition than developed condition. The three methods of treatment are:

- *Open reduction:* This could lead to a painful hip at a later stage.
- *Osteotomy of the proximal femur:* This has been tried with varying results.
- THR in late cases.

CENTRAL DISLOCATION OF HIP

This is the least common and most difficult of all dislocations of the hip joint.

Table 4.1 gives a comparative study of the various types of dislocations of the hip joint.

Mechanism of Injury

It could be due to direct blow on the greater trochanter as in the case of RTA or fall on the sides (Fig. 4.17). It is invariably associated with the fractures of the acetabulum and this is what makes it a very difficult problem to treat.

Classification: Judet's Types

- Undisplaced fractures (Either single-line or stellate types).
- *Inner wall fractures*
  - Femoral head concentrically reduced beneath the dome on initial X-rays.
  - Femoral head not reduced under the acetabular dome but centrally dislocated.
- *Superior dome fractures*
  - Gross outline of the acetabular dome intact and congruous with the femoral head.

Table 4.1: Comparative features of dislocations of hip

	Posterior dislocation	*Anterior dislocation*	*Central dislocation*
Incidence	Common (70%)	10–15%	Rare
Mechanism of injury	• Dashboard injury as in RTA • Flexed knee + neutral adduction results in simple dislocation. • Flexed knee + slight abduction results in fracture dislocation	• Dashboard injury with thigh abducted • Fall from height • Blow to the back in squatted position	• Due to direct blow over trochanter • Common in patients with epilepsy, convulsions, etc.
Classification	*Thompson and Epstein* • *Type I* with or without minor fracture • *Type II* with a large single fracture of rim acetabulum • *Type III* comminution of acetabular rim with or without major fragment. • *Type IV* with fracture of femoral head	*Type I* (Superior) • *IA* No fracture • *IB* Associated head fracture • *IC* Associated fracture acetabulum *Type II* (Inferior) • *IIA* No fracture • *IIB* Associated head fracture • *IIC* Associated fracture acetabulum	*Judet's* Dislocation associated with • Undisplaced fracture • Inner wall fracture of acetabulum • Superior rim fracture of acetabulum • Bursting fracture of acetabulum
Clinical features	• Limb shortening • Flexion/add/IR deformity • Thigh rests on the contralateral limb • Head felt in the gluteal region • Vascular sign-ve (Narath) • Movements of hip ↓ • Injury to sciatic nerve	*Superior type* flexion + abd + external rotation deformity *Inferior type* hip is extended and externally rotated • Head felt superiorly or inferiorly • Vascular sign (Narath) +ve • Injury to femoral nerve artery or vein	• No limb shortening • Limb is neutral in position • Bruising over the greater trochanter • Per rectal examination reveals head of femur

Contd.

Table 4.1: Comparative features of dislocations of hip *(Contd.)*

	Posterior dislocation	*Anterior dislocation*	*Central dislocation*
Treatment	*Four Methods of Closed Reduction* 1. *Stimson's gravity method:* Least traumatic but associated injuries prevent prone positioning 2. *Allis:* Traction is given in line of deformity 3. *Bigelow's method:* Reduction is done by causing the opposite methods of ext/abd/ER 4. *Classical Watson-Jones method:* Limb is brought to the neutral position first then longitudinal traction in the line of femur is given.	1. *Stimson's gravity method* 2. *Allis method* 3. *Reverse Bigelow's method:* Here position of hip is flexion and adduction 4. *Classical method:* It is as described for posterior dislocation	Reduction is attempted through skeletal traction on greater trochanter in line of the neck of femur. If it fails, open reduction is indicated
Complications	*Early* • Sciatic nerve palsy • Irreducible fracture dislocation • Missed knee injuries • Recurrent dislocations *Late* • Myositis ossificans • Avascular necrosis of bone • Post-traumatic arthritis • Unreduced posterior dislocation	*Early* • Neurovascular injuries • Femoral artery, vein, nerve injury • Irreducibility *Late* • Post-traumatic osteoarthritis • Aseptic necrosis • Recurrent dislocation	*I Early* • Sciatic nerve palsy • Superior gluteal artery injury • Bowel obstruction • Thrombophlebitis • Infection • Recurrent dislocation *II Late* • Post-traumatic arthritis • AVN • Nonunion • Myositis ossificans

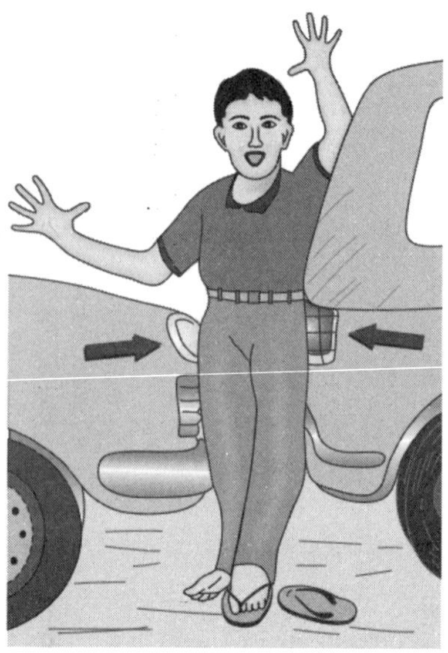

Fig. 4.17: Common mechanism of central dislocation of the hip

  - Gross outline of the acetabular dome not intact and not congruous with the femoral head.
- Bursting fractures (All elements of the acetabulum are involved)
  - Fractures in which congruity remains between the femoral head and acetabular dome.
  - Fractures in which there is incongruity between the femoral head and acetabular dome.

Clinical Features

Interestingly none of the features as in ADH or PDH is seen. On the other hand, in CDH there is no limb shortening, no external rotation deformity, head is not externally palpable. The limb is in neutral position; there is pain, severe restriction of hip movements and a huge bruise over the greater trochanter. Head is felt easily by a per-rectal examination.

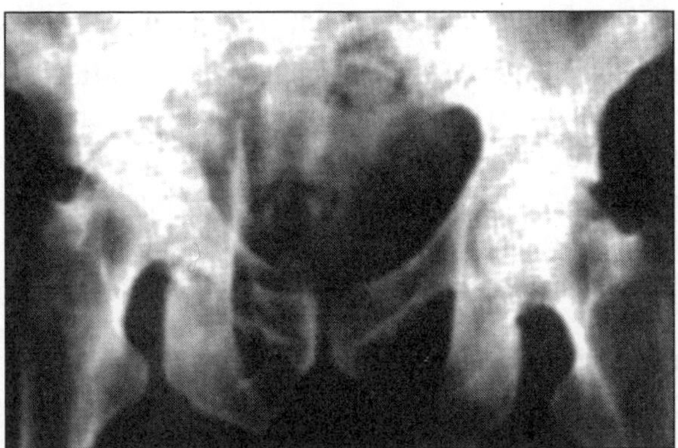

Fig. 4.18: Radiograph showing central fracture dislocation of the hip joint

Investigations

X-ray evaluation: Plain X-ray plays a very important role in the diagnosis of these injuries (Fig. 4.18). The recommended views are AP view of the pelvis, internal and external oblique views. The former view helps in the demonstration of the femoral head acetabular relationship while the latter views helps in delineating fracture lines and displacement.

CT scan: This helps to delineate the fracture lines better and with far more great accuracy than plain X-rays.

MRI scan: This helps to study the vascularity of the femoral head and the bony and cartilage architecture.

Treatment: Reduction of the dislocation assumes lot of clinical importance, as it is essential to obtain as accurate a reduction as possible to restore the acetabular congruity. This helps prevent post-traumatic osteoarthritis.

- *Skeletal traction:* Reduction is achieved through skeletal traction over the greater trochanter in line of the neck of femur. Open reduction is reserved for cases of failed closed reduction. The skeletal traction is maintained for 10–12 weeks if the acetabulum is reasonably reconstructed.

- *Open reduction and internal fixation:* If the reconstruction of the acetabulum is far from satisfactory, after the mandatory skeletal traction, then open reduction and surgical reconstruction of the acetabulum is recommended.
- *Primary arthroplasty or arthrodesis:* This is recommended in extreme cases where closed reduction fails and open reduction reveals severe articular damage.

Complications

Early complications: This includes sciatic nerve palsy, superior gluteal artery injury, thrombophlebitis, bowel obstruction, aseptic necrosis, pin-tract infection, recurrent central dislocations, etc.

Delayed complications: Post-traumatic osteoarthritis is an escapable complication in central dislocation. Other fearful complications include myositis, avascular necrosis of the femoral head and a stiff and disabling hip.

5 Injuries Around the Hip—Fractures of Neck Femur

UPPER OR PROXIMAL FEMORAL FRACTURES

Upper part of femur is called proximal femoral fractures and this includes fracture neck of femur and trochanteric fractures and are discussed below.

FRACTURE NECK OF FEMUR

Quotation: We come to the world under the brim of pelvis and go out of the world through the fracture neck of femur. This indicates the gravity of this fracture. In earlier times it invariably meant death. Hence this saying.

Types of Neck Fractures

Fracture neck femur could be intracapsular or extracapsular. Intracapsular fracture neck femur is notoriously known as an orthopedic enigma, since a permanent solution for its treatment still eludes the orthopedic surgeon. Hence, it is infamously termed as an unsolved problem. Fracture neck of femur does not unite readily and this makes it a difficult problem to tackle (*see* box for the reasons).

Problems of healing, why?

- No cambium layer in the intracapsular area, so no peripheral callus. Healing is only by endosteal callus.
- Synovial fluid lyses blood clot at the fracture site and thereby destroys another mode of secondary healing.
- Displaced fracture leads to avascularity.

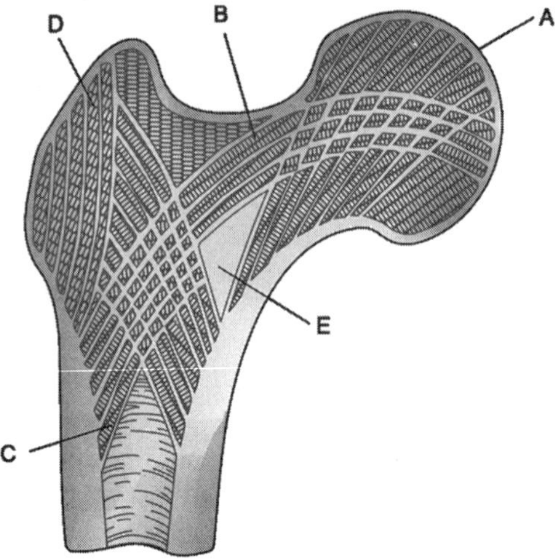

Fig. 5.1: Trabecular pattern or proximal femur: (A) Primary compressive trabeculae, (B) Primary tensile trabeculae, (C) Secondary tensile, (D) Secondary compressive trabeculae, (E) Ward's triangle

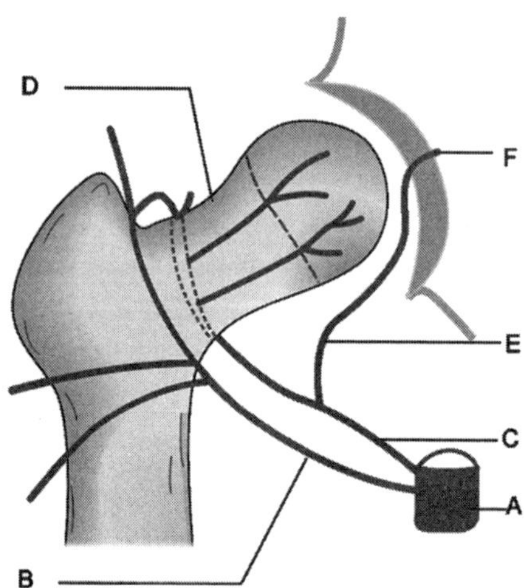

Fig. 5.2: Vascular anatomy of femoral head: (A) Profunda femoris artery, (B) Lateral circumflex artery, (C) Medial circumflex artery, (D) Ascending retinacular vessels, (E) Obturator branch of medial circumflex artery, (F) Artery of the ligamentum teres

Why hip fractures are a dreaded problem?

The answer for this difficult question lies in its peculiar blood supply. Here are the technical details about the precarious vascular supply.

Vascular Anatomy and its Significance

Avascular necrosis of femoral head and nonunion fracture neck femur are the two very important and common complications of intracapsular fracture neck femur. A thorough knowledge of the vascular anatomy (Fig. 5.2) is necessary to understand the reasons behind. Femoral head circulation is through three sources:

- Intraosseous cervical vessels.
- Artery of ligamentum teres.
- Retinacular vessels.

In fracture neck femur, intraosseous cervical vessels are disrupted and blood supply is dependent on artery of ligamentum teres and retinacular vessels only. Artery of ligamentum teres supplies only a small portion of head, hence, avascular necrosis of the head of the femur occurs if retinacular vessels, the only main source, are damaged in fracture neck femur. There are two sources of viability of femoral head after a displaced femoral neck fracture:

1. Residual uninjured vascular supply.
2. Revascularization of neck of femur from surrounding soft tissue before late segmental collapse.

"Therefore, the aim of treatment is early anatomical reduction, impaction and rigid internal fixation to protect the existing circulation and to allow revascularization to take place before late segmental collapse can occur."

In whom it is common? Etiology

- It is common in older patients with osteoporosis or osteomalacia (12%) and in them usually it is fracture through a weak pathological bone.

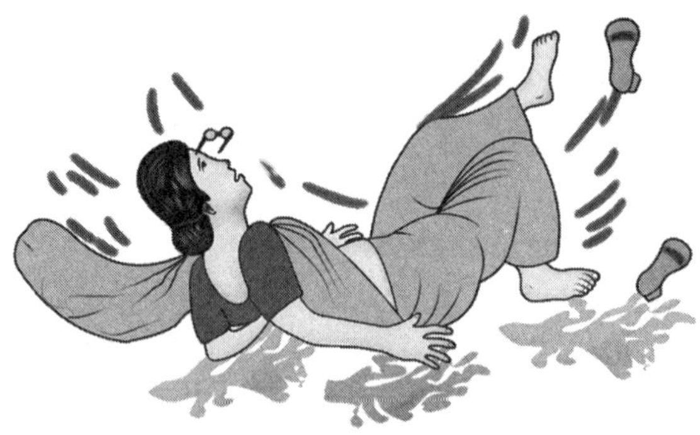

Fig. 5.3: Fracture neck femur is common in elderly females due to trivial fall like a slip and fall in the bathroom

- It is common in elderly women secondary to senile osteoporosis. It also causes marked comminution of the posterior cortex and thus decreases the quality of reduction.

How is this injury caused? Mechanism of injury

- Majority of the neck fractures are due to trivial fall, because of the impact of the direct blow over the greater trochanter (Fig. 5.3).
- Second mechanism is mainly due to lateral rotation of the extremity, which causes marked posterior comminution of the neck.
- Recent suggested mechanism is cyclical loading due to muscle force and torsion.
- Major trauma in young adults like road traffic accident (RTA), fall, etc.

What are the nature of these fractures? Classification

Many classifications are proposed for fracture neck femur. This is important to identify the various types of fractures of the neck femur and the best possible treatment options for the same. Few important classification ones are mentioned here for the benefit of the medical students and is named after the pioneers who described them.

Broad Classification

- Intracapsular fracture—from subcapital area to the middle of the neck.
- Extracapsular fracture —from base of the neck to the pertrochanteric region (Fig. 5.4).

Structural Classification

- Impacted fracture—here the fragments are telescoped into each other.
- Undisplaced fracture.
- Displaced fracture.

Causatively

- Stress fractures (seen in soldiers, athletes, etc.)
- Pathologic fractures (seen in osteoporosis, etc.)
- Post-irradiation fractures.

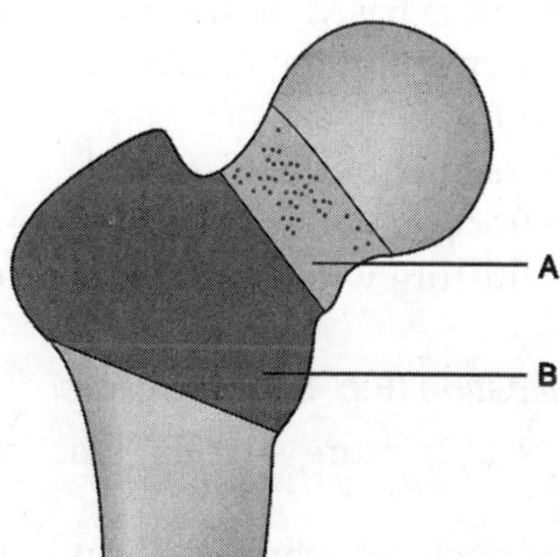

Fig. 5.4: Fracture neck femur types: (A) Intracapsular region, and (B) Extracapsular region

Based on Fracture Characters

- *Anatomical location:*
  - Subcapital fracture—beneath the neck.
  - Transcervical fracture—in the middle of the neck.
  - Basal—at the base of the neck.
- Bank's subclassification
  - Classical subcapital
  - Wedge subcapital (common)
  - Inferior beak appearance.
- Based on the *fracture angles:*
  - Pauwel's (angle the fracture line forms with respect to horizontal line Fig. 5.5).

  More the angle more is it likely to be unstable.
  - I 30°
  - II 50°
  - III 70°
    - Perlington's (angle the fracture line forms with respect to the vertical line)
  - I 70°
  - II 50°
  - III 30°
- Garden's classification (Fig. 5.6) This is the most accepted classification and is based on the pattern of fracture line and the displacement of the fracture:
  - Incomplete fracture
  - Complete fracture but undisplaced
  - Complete fracture with partial displacement
  - Complete fracture with total displacement.

Delbet's Classification (Fig. 5.7) *in Children*

- Transepiphyseal fracture —at the junction of the head and neck.
- Transcervical fracture —through the middle of the neck.
- Cervicotrochanteric fracture (basal) at the junction of neck and shaft.

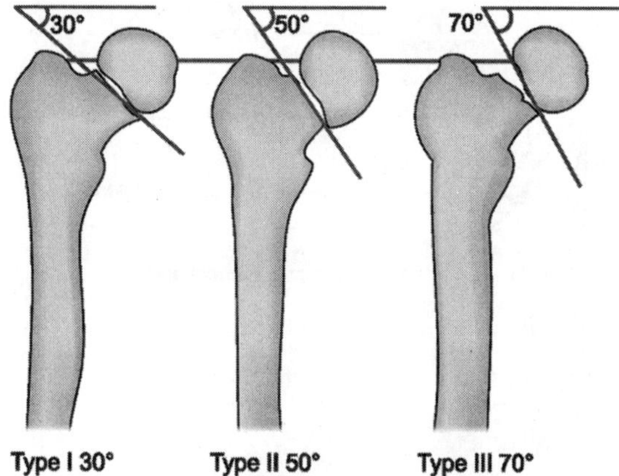

Fig. 5.5: Pauwel's classification of fracture neck femur

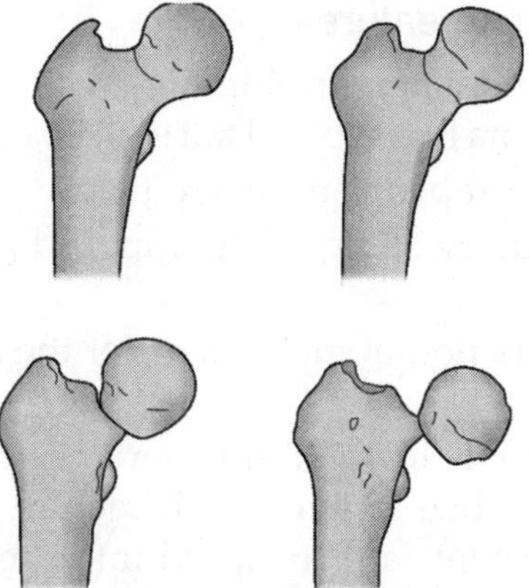

Fig. 5.6: Garden's classification

- Intertrochanteric fracture in between the greater and lesser trochanters.
- Pertrochanteric fracture —at the level of the trochanter.

> ***Note:*** Garden and Pauwel's classification in adults and Delbet's classification in children are widely used while the others are mentioned for student's information.

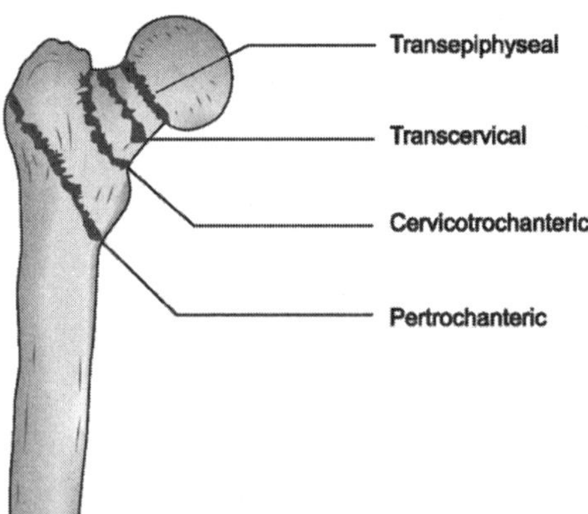

Fig. 5.7: Delbet's classification for fracture neck of femur in children

How does a patient with fracture neck of femur present? Clinical features

- Usually, the patient is an elderly female and gives history of trivial trauma like slip and fall in the bathroom (Fig. 5.3).
- The patient complains of severe pain.
- There may be swelling of the hip and over the greater trochanter.
- There is restriction of movements of the affected hip.

On examination

- Patient is unable to walk in majority of the cases. But in rare instances like an impacted fracture where both the fracture fragments are collapsed into each other, patient may walk with pain and limp.
- There is severe tenderness over the anterior hip joint line.
- There is minimal shortening and external rotational deformity of the affected limb due to the fracture being intracapsular. The capsule prevents the muscular forces from displacing the fracture fragments grossly.
- Active straight leg rising is difficult.
- In impacted fracture neck of femur, the patient complains of groin pain, antalgic gait and restriction of hip movements.

Investigations

Radiography

This consists of routine plain X-rays including AP and lateral views of the hip joint. The following points are noted on the X-rays (Fig. 5.8).

- The extent of fracture line whether complete or incomplete
- The fracture angle.
- Break in the *Shenton's line* (Fig. 5.9). *Shenton's line* is a line drawn from the superior margin of the obturator foramen to the margin of the neck.

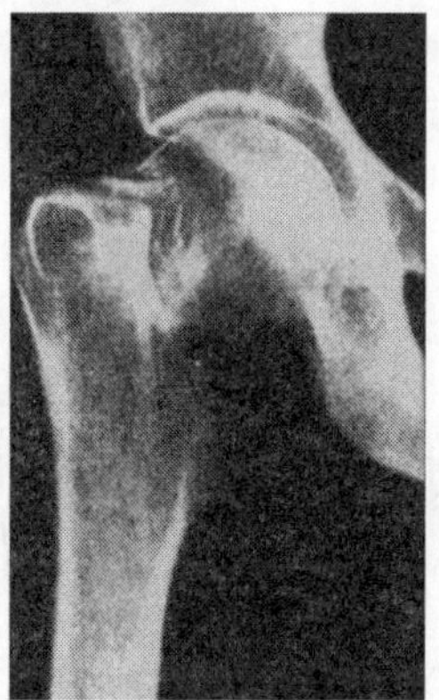

Fig. 5.8: Radiograph showing intracapsular, e.g. fracture neck femur

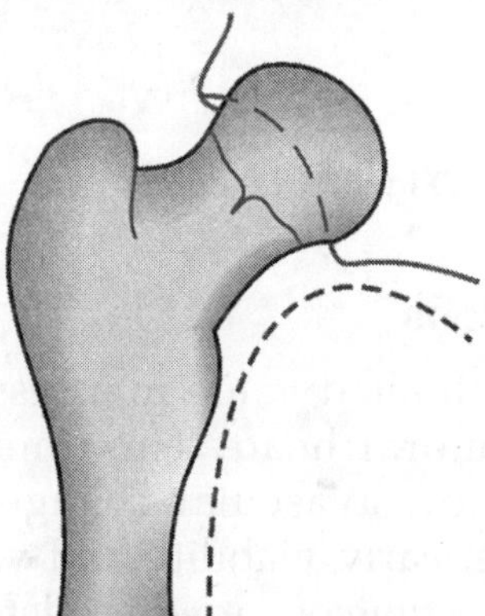

Fig. 5.9: Shenton's line

- Posterior wall comminution of the neck is best seen in the lateral view.
- Prominent lesser trochanter.
- *Singh's index:* This classification system measures the degree of osteoporosis in the proximal femur based on radiographic evaluation of the trabecular pattern of the proximal femur (Fig. 5.10). This helps to decide the choice of implants.

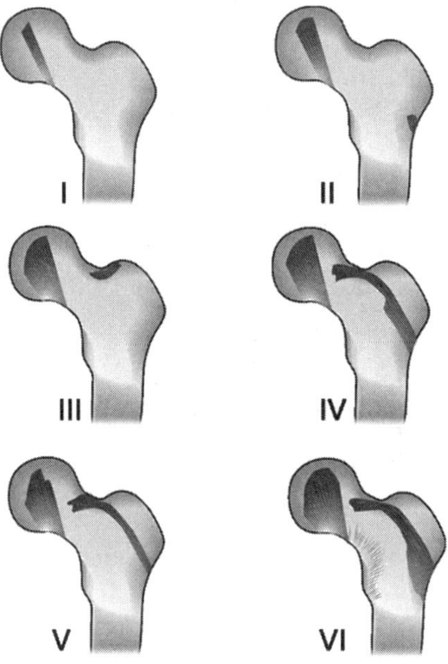

Fig. 5.10: Singh's index

Other Investigations

Radiography has limited value in assessing the vascular status of the femoral head. The time required for a radiograph to show avascular changes is 3–6 months (Fig. 5.11). Hence, early viability and vascularization of femoral head at the time of surgery is determined by:

- Oxygen tension measurement

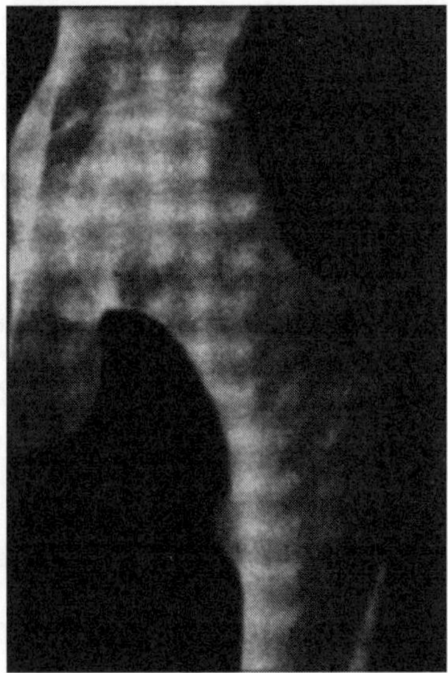

Fig. 5.11: Radiograph showing avascular necrosis of femoral head

- Venography
- Intraosseous pressure recording
- Isotope scanning
- Bone scan with technetium-99m, sulphur colloid, etc.

How to treat fracture neck of femur? Treatment

Fracture neck femur is an orthopedic emergency, which needs to be reduced and fixed within 24 hours to get an optimum result. Hence, *speed is the watchword* in managing fracture neck femur and invariably needs to be operated and because of the small proximal fragment accurate reduction is required, which is usually not possible by conservative methods.

Aims of Treatment

- Early anatomical reduction, which helps and prevents further vascular damage.
- Impaction of the fracture fragments.

- *Rigid internal fixation:* This enables revascularization from the surrounding soft tissues and uninjured bones, which helps in early callus formation.

Broad treatment guidelines (Earlier)

Age group	Undisplaced	Displaced
>70 years	• Dynamic hip Screws (DHS)	• Prosthesis • Total hip replacement (THR)
Young adults	• DHS • Cannulated screws (ASNIS)	• DHS • Later osteotomy or prosthesis
Children	• HIP spica • Multiple Moore's pinning	• Multiple Moore's pinning • Osteotomy • Arthrodesis

Broad treatment guidelines for displaced neck fracture (Now)

- < 65 years—CRIF/Or ORIF if necessary
- 65–75 years—CRIF and if closed reduction is unsuccessful then cemented bipolar arthroplasty.
- >75 years—Cemented bipolar arthroplasty
- >75 years (and poor home ambulator)—cemented unipolar arthroplasty
- >75 years (bedridden)—Percutaneous CRIF under local or sedation
- Persistent arthritis—Total hip replacement
- Bed ridden and not mobile—Nonoperative or CRIF

Broad Treatment Plans as per Garden's Classification

Garden I

- Conservative Hip spica is applied if fracture is several weeks old and if the patient is unfit for surgery.
- Surgical Multiple pins by Moore, Knowles cannulated screws, etc.

Garden II: Here the fracture is complete and may be displaced. Hence, it is fixed with either DHS or multiple cannulated AO screws.

Garden III/IV: Conservative treatment is rarely indicated except in severely ill patients and mentally ill patients, e.g. hip spica and well leg traction. Surgery is the treatment of choice.

Surgery: Barring a few cases like impacted fractures, surgery in the treatment of choice in these fractures.

Goal of surgery

- Anatomical reduction
- Impaction
- Stable internal fixation

In displaced fractures, one needs to reduce the fracture first before fixing it? Reduction techniques

Reduction technique could be closed or open. Whatever is the technique, acceptable reduction is the key factor in decreasing risk of avascular necrosis following fracture neck femur. Closed reduction is tried first failing which open reduction is resorted to. The following are the closed reduction methods

Closed reduction with hip in extension	*Closed reduction with hip in flexion*
Whitman's method Extension + internal rotation + abduction Movements of the hip	**Lead better method** Flexion of hip, traction along long axis of femur, thigh internally rotated and abducted. Evaluate reduction by *"heel palm test".
Massie Forceful internal rotation of the limb	**Smith Peterson** Slight hip flexion + then internal rotation + abduction + extension
Mc Elevenny Extension + external Rotation + Internal Rotation + adduction movements	**Flynn** Flexion, traction along the femoral neck
Deyerle Traction with extension + foot is internally rotated + Force applied on greater trochanter from anterior to posterior direction	

*What is 'heel palm' test? It is a clinical test to assess the accuracy of reduction of fracture neck femur. The heel of the affected limb should remain neutral in the palm of the clinician's hand and not lie externally rotated after reduction.

How to assess the accuracy of the fracture reduction?

Radiographic evaluation of the accuracy of reduction of the fracture neck femur, obtained by any one of the reduction methods mentioned above is done. It is mandatory before proceeding with internal fixation. The following are some of the parameters:

- Head and neck always form an S-shaped curve. If the radiograph reveals an unbroken C-shaped curve the fracture is not reduced.
- *Garden's criteria:* In AP view, normal alignment index between proximal and distal fragments post-reduction is 155–180°.

  In lateral view, it is 160–180°. If the angle is less than 155° or more than 180° in of the views, then the reduction is not acceptable.
- *Lateral view* helps to detect the posterior wall comminution. Stability of reduction depends on posterior wall comminution, which causes nonunion in 60 percent of the cases.
- Slight valgus with 2–3 mm separation of the fracture site at the medial calcar is not acceptable. However, varus is not accepted at all.

Caution: If two attempts at closed reduction fail, then open reduction is resorted to. Probably, there is no other fracture, which needs such an accurate reduction before proceeding for internal fixation. Hence, the reduction should be accurately assessed to get good results.

What are the Techniques of Internal Fixation for the Fracture Neck of Femur?

Once the fracture needs to be fixed, what are the fixation options before the surgeon? There are many choices for internal fixation in fracture neck femur, but the principles of preoperative preparation, reduction of the fracture, C-arm or radiographic control, surgical approaches and methods of insertion of fixations are the same.

Procedure of internal fixation

- The patient is fixed to the fracture table after anesthesia.
- Closed reduction of the fracture is done under radiograph or C-arm control.
- If the reduction is satisfactory, the greater trochanter and upper end of femur is exposed through a lateral incision.
- Midway between the anterior and posterior cortices of the lateral femur and about 2 cm distal to the edge of the greater trochanter drill a hole, insert a guide pin at an angle of 45° to the shaft, and parallel to the ground.
- Check the positions of the guide-wires by lateral radiographs or C-arm. If satisfactory, insert the cannulated screws or Moore's pins parallel to the guide-wire and if Richard's screw is used through the guide-wire.
- Confirm the position of all the pins as mentioned above and close the wound in layers. Postoperatively, the patient is mobilized early.

Choices of Implants for Internal Fixation

After having accurately reduced the fracture and ascertained the accuracy, the fracture neck femur can be fixed by any one of the methods mentioned below. However, no ideal internal fixation methods are available (Figs 5.12A to C).

- *Multiple Pins (Knowles, Moore)* for impacted fracture, percutaneously for medically unfit persons, and for fractures in children (Fig. 5.12D).
- *ASNIS:* This is a system of cannulated screws that provide improved pullout and bending and torque strengths as compared to Knowles pins. These are the commonly preferred screws for the intracapsular variety.
- *Fixed angle nail* has fallen into disrepute because the nail is rigid and may penetrate the joint (Fig. 5.12B).

- *Sliding or telescoping nails (dynamic hip screws):* It has replaced the fixed angle nail. The nail offers collapsibility which ensures continuous impaction at the fracture site and which lessens the chance of nail penetration through the femoral head. This is the most commonly employed fixation method for fracture neck femur, especially the extracapsular variety (Fig. 5.12C).

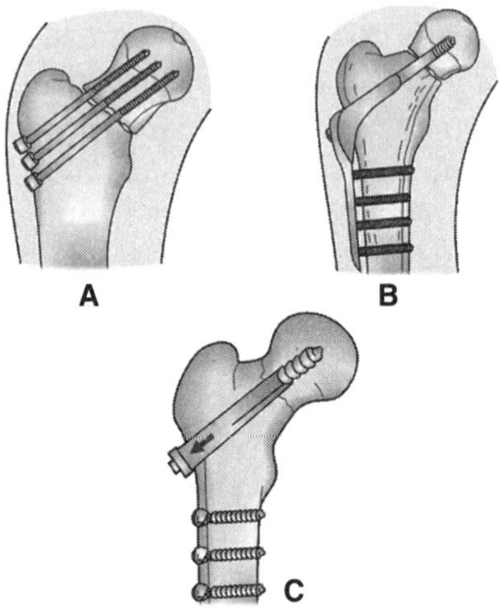

Figs 5.12A to C: Methods of internal fixation of intracapsular fracture neck of femur: (A) Multiple pins, (B) Blade plate fixation, (C) Dynamic hip screw

Cardinal Points in Internal Fixation

- Guide-pin should be inserted at an angle of 45° to the shaft and parallel to the ground.
- Guide-pin should be in the center and stop short of the head by 1.3 cm.
- The internal fixation screws or pins should be in the mid-center of the neck or below and posterior to prevent damage to the retinacular vessels.
- The guide-pin should be inserted slowly and should pass smoothly without any resistance.

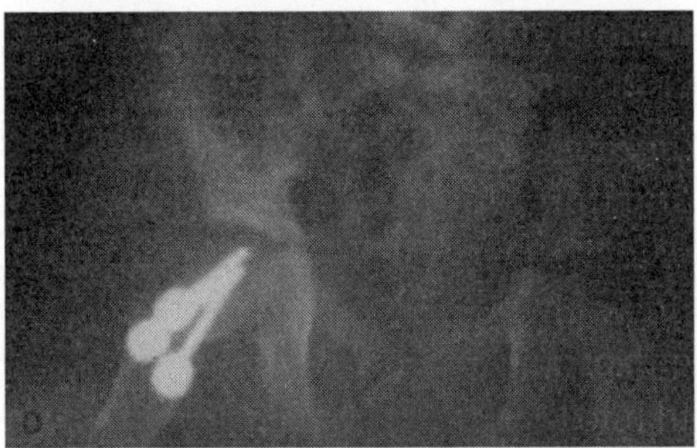

Fig. 5.12D: Fixation with multiple Moore's pin in children

- The screws or pins should be 0.6 cm shorter when placed above and 0.6 cm longer when placed below the guide-pin.

Complications of Internal Fixation

Infection: This is due to poor aseptic measures during surgery. The infection may be superficial or deep and is a troublesome problem to treat.

Nonunion results if the fixation methods are not rigid.

Avascular necrosis: This is due to faulty position of the pins in the superior part of the neck, which may damage the retinacular vessels leading to avascularity.

Loss of fixation: This could occur due to osteoporosis, loosening, etc.

Meyer's Muscle Pedicle Graft

A mention has to be made about the posterior muscle pedicle grafting technique. Muscle pedicle graft from the gluteus maximus or quadratus femoris (Meyer's technique), is particularly useful in posterior wall comminution. Dr Bakshi of Kolkata has popularized this technique.

Other Treatment Options

These include hemireplacement arthroplasty, osteotomy and very rarely total hip replacement (THR). However, they are not recommended as the primary modality of treatment in fresh fracture neck of femur. They are indicated in special situations like nonunion, AVN, etc. and are discussed below.

But however, hemireplacement arthroplasty or THR as a primary treatment in displaced intracapsular fracture neck of femur over 70 years is a better option than internal fixation except in very frail patients where internal fixation seem to do better. When compared to fixation techniques, primary prosthetic replacement preferably with a bipolar prosthesis allows for immediate weight bearing, eliminates the chances of AVN and nonunion and has reduced chances of re-surgery later.

Now *bipolar arthroplasty* has largely replaced the unipolar arthroplasty of yesteryears (Austin and Thompson's prosthesis) as this eliminates the complication of protrusio acetabuli which may be associated with unipolar prosthesis.

However, after 70 years, in displaced fracture of femoral neck, amongst the treatment options of internal fixation, hemireplacement arthroplasty and THR, THR seems to be the best bet with lower complications.

THIS IS WHY FRACTURE NECK OF FEMUR IS DREADED PROBLEM DUE TO ITS COMPLICATIONS

Thromboembolism

Thromboembolism is a leading cause of death within first 7 days. Incidence is 40 percent and needs to be identified and tackled early to prevent mortality.

Nonunion

Despite the best efforts only one-third of the fracture neck femur are known to heal with OR + IF. Nonunion rate is 85–95 percent. If there is no evidence of radiological healing taking place between 6 and 12 months at treatment on a radiograph, it is declared as nonunion.

Why do fracture neck of the femur fail to unite? Causes

a. Inaccurate reduction.
b. Poor internal fixation.
c. Lack of cambium layer in the periosteum of the neck.
d. Avascularity of femoral head.
e. Posterior wall comminution.

How does the patient present? Clinical features

- The patient complains of pain.
- The patient is unable to bear the weight on the affected side.
- Movements of the hip are affected.
- If the patient manages to walk, there could be limp.
- Trendelenburg test, telescopic test will be positive.
- Wasting of the muscles and
- Minimal shortening of the affected lower limb are the other features.

Radiograph

Plain radiographs of the hip reveal ununited fracture neck of femur and there may be avascular changes in the head and in very late cases, secondary osteoarthritis of the hip joint (Fig. 5.13).

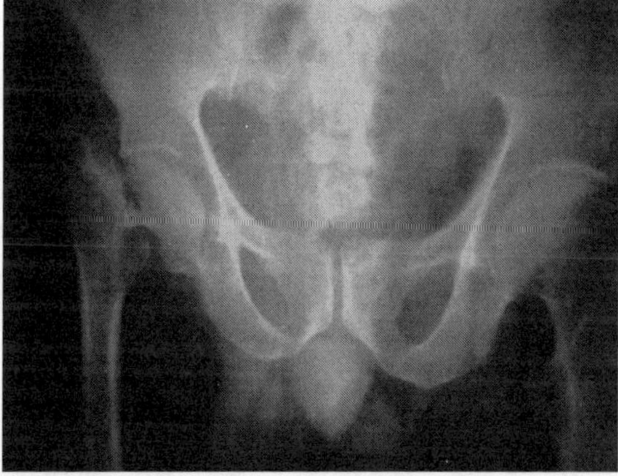

Fig. 5.13: Radiograph showing nonunion fracture neck of femur

How does one manage this dreaded complication?
Treatment

For nonunion fracture neck of femur, surgery is the treatment of choice. The method chosen takes into account the viability of the head.

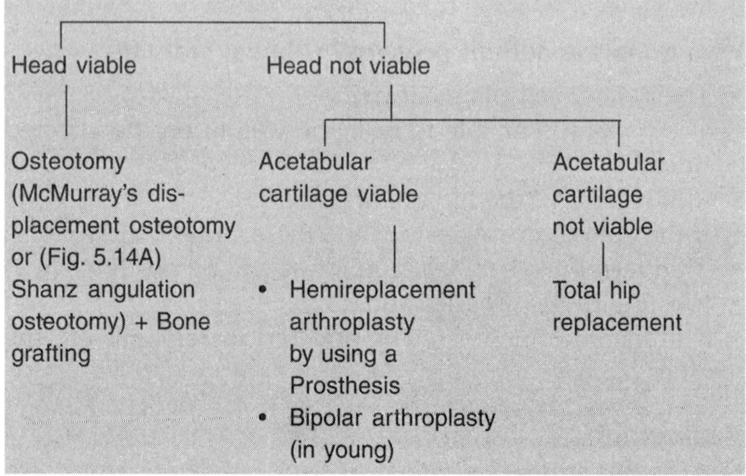

Osteotomy

Osteotomy as a treatment for nonunion fracture neck femur has a role only if the head of the femur is viable otherwise, hemiarthroplasty is preferable.

To treat nonunion of fracture neck femur, two types of osteotomies and their modifications have been described and they are as follows:

McMurray's displacement osteotomy: In this, the osteotomy is made just proximal to the lesser trochanter and the distal fragment is pushed medially and fixed internally (Fig. 5.14A).

Shanz angulation osteotomy: In this, the osteotomy is made through or just distal to the lesser trochanter. A laterally based wedge of bone is removed and the varus angulation is corrected and fixed with plate and screws (Fig. 5.14B).

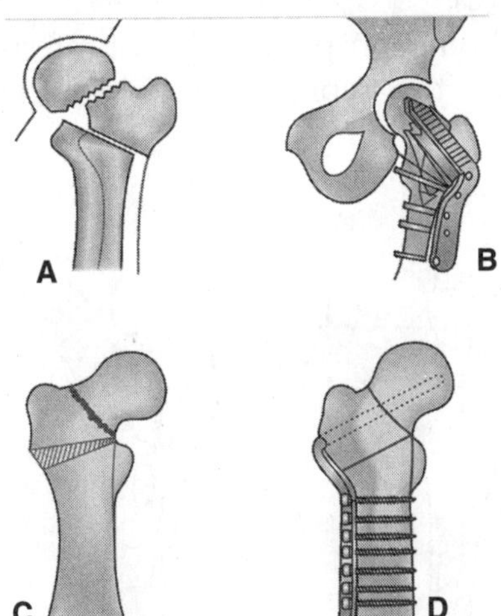

Figs 5.14A to D: Different types of osteotomies: (A) McMurray's osteotomy, (B) Shanz angulation osteotomy, (C) Angulation osteotomy, (D) Pauwel's osteotomy

What is the Role of Osteotomy?

Displacement or angulation osteotomy helps to convert the shearing force at the fracture site into compression forces by changing the line of weight bearing and thereby enhances the chances of fracture union (Figs 5.14C and D).

Among the two, angulation osteotomy is preferable because the position of greater trochanter is more satisfactory, function of the abductor muscles is re-established more effectively, there is no further shortening and internal fixation is maintained more satisfactorily.

Hemireplacement Arthroplasty

As mentioned earlier, if the head is not viable but the acetabular cartilage is viable, and if the patient is over 60 years of age, hemireplacement arthroplasty is the treatment of choice. However, the choice of prosthesis depends upon the existing calcar femori. If sufficiently present (at least 1-3 cm), Austin Moore's prosthesis is the choice and if it is inadequate, Thompson prosthesis is preferred (Figs 5.15A and B). Bipolar hip replacement is another option (Fig. 5.16).

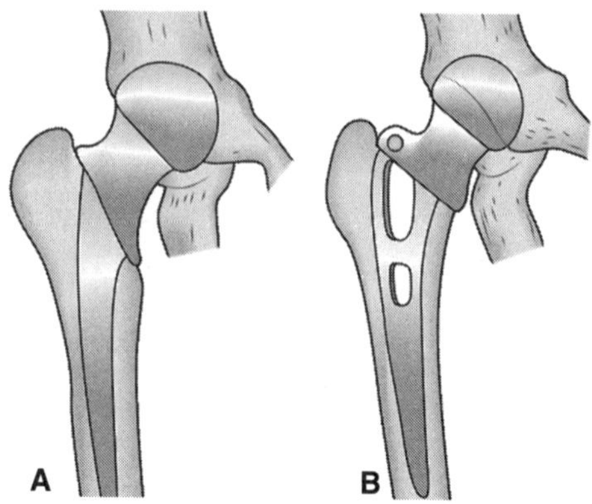

Figs 5.15A and B: Types of hemireplacement arthroplasty: (A) Thompson's prosthesis, and (B) Austin Moore's prosthesis

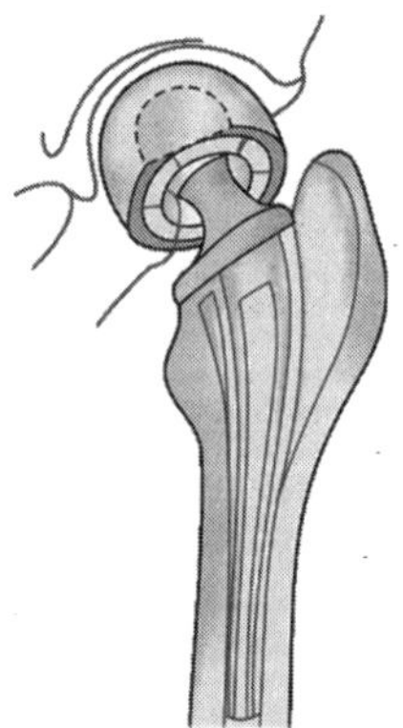

Fig. 5.16: Bipolar arthroplasty

Total Hip Replacement

If both the femoral head and the acetabular cartilage is not viable and if the patient is more than 60 years old total hip replacement is the surgery of choice.

Avascular Necrosis

It is the next important complication. Two types are described:

- *Due to actual AVN:* This is secondary to ischemia and is an early phenomenon. It shows characteristic microscopic appearance.
- *Late segmental collapse:* It is due to collapse of subchondral and articular cartilage that overlies infarcted bone. It occurs late.

Incidence

- *Aseptic necrosis* 66–84 percent.
- *Late segmental collapse* 7–27 percent.

In displaced femoral neck fracture, femoral head survival is dependent on vessels of ligamentum teres which is absent in one-third cases and subfoveal artery anastomosis which is variable and incomplete. All vessels within femoral neck and most of the retinacular vessels are disrupted in displaced fracture. Hence, survival of head depends on:

- Uninjured vascular supply
- Revascularization: *Vascular injury occurs*
  a. at the time of fracture commonly.
  b. during reduction or internal fixation.

Hence, good anatomical reduction and stable internal fixation is required to preserve the remaining blood supply, which helps in revascularization.

Investigations

Plain radiographs of the hip joint shows increased density of the femoral head, and this may take 6 months to 2 years to be seen on radiograph (Fig. 5.8). In late cases, there may be secondary osteoarthritis changes within the hip joint.

Bone scan: by this early and accurate determination of avascularity can be made, but it is not 100 percent accurate.

Treatment of AVN is by no means easy. Here are the options

- Symptomatic treatment like bed rest, non-steroidal anti-inflammatory drugs (NSAIDs), etc.
- Displacement or angulation osteotomy in early stages.
- If acetabular cartilage is viable, hemireplacement prosthesis is preferred.
- Total hip replacement if acetabular cartilage is not viable.

Quick Recap: Fracture neck of femur at a glance

- An unsolved problem.
- Fracture of the elderly.
- Majority due to trivial fall.
- Garden's classification widely accepted.
- It is an orthopedic emergency.
- Speed is the watchword in management.
- Early anatomical reduction, impaction, and rigid internal fixation are the aim of treatment.
- DHS and multiple cannulated cancellous screws is the currently accepted method of fixation.
- Nonunion and AVN are very common.

TROCHANTERIC FRACTURE

Salient Features

- An intertrochanteric fracture occurs along a line between greater trochanter and lesser trochanter with variable comminution (Fig. 5.17).
- Totally extracapsular.
- Internal rotators of the hip remain attached to the distal fragment; short external rotators are attached to proximal head and neck. Hence, limb has to be kept in external rotation after reduction to align the distal fragment with proximal one.
- Cancellous bone heals well by 8–12 weeks.
- Four times more common than intracapsular fracture.

Age: Seen in elderly patients 10–12 years older than intracapsular fracture neck femur.

Sex: More common in females (2.8:1).

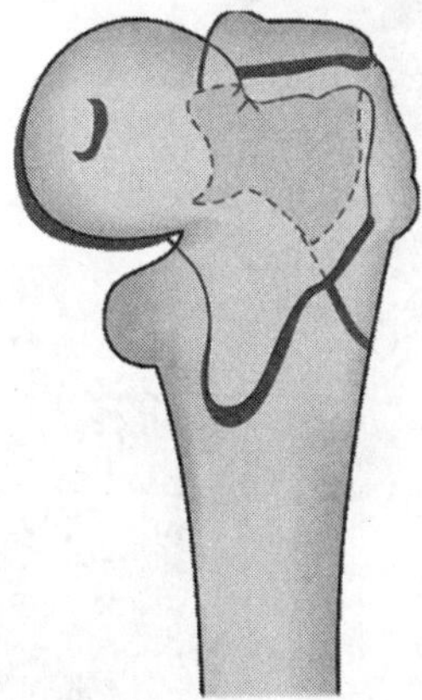

Fig. 5.17: Comminuted intertrochanteric fracture

Mechanism

Direct trauma to the trochanter as in RTA, fall, etc.

Indirect trauma due to violent muscle pull, etc.

What are the Clinical Features?

The patient unlike in fracture neck of femur will have
- Marked pain
- Marked shortening of the lower limb
- Complete external rotation deformity
- Gross swelling
- Ecchymosis and
- Tenderness over the greater trochanter.

Radiograph

A true anteroposterior view in internal rotation and a lateral view help to study the fracture pattern (Fig. 5.18).

How to manage these fractures? Treatment

Conservative treatment: There is 10 percent mortality associated with conservative treatment of this fracture.

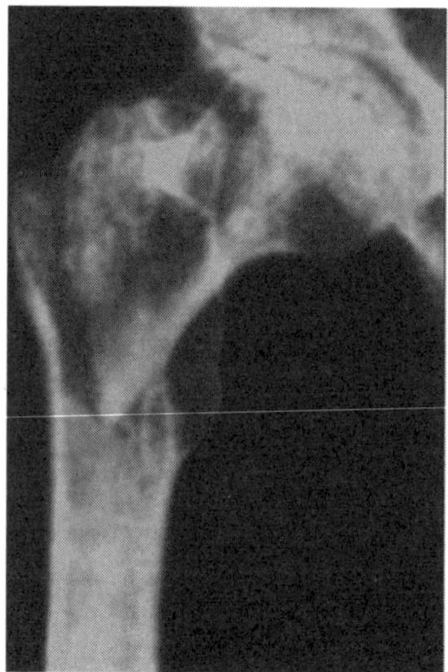

Fig. 5.18: Radiograph showing comminuted trochanteric fracture femur

Indications

- Poor medical and surgical risk patients.
- Terminally ill patients.
- Very old patients.

Methods

- Simple support with pillows
- Buck's traction
- Plaster spica
- Skeletal traction through distal femur or tibia for 10–12 weeks (Fig. 5.19).

Surgical: Though not an emergency, there is an urgent need for surgery as there is a 10-fold increase in mortality, if surgery is delayed for more than 48 hours.

Advantages of surgery include increased comfort, good nursing care and hospitalization stay is considerably reduced.

Goal is to fix a stably reduced fracture internally.

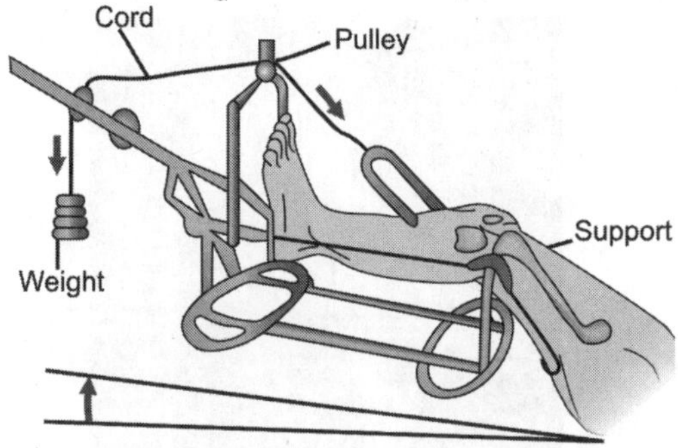

Fig. 5.19: Skeletal traction through Böhler-Braun frame for trochanteric fracture

Reduce the fracture before fixing it is the mantra

Methods of Reduction

Closed reduction is by traction, slight abduction and external rotation. If proper reduction is not obtained by this method, then open reduction is done.

Open Reduction Option

Indications:

- Failed closed reduction.
- Large spike on proximal fragment with lesser trochanter intact.
- Reverse oblique fracture.

Choice of an Implant

Once stable reduction has been obtained either anatomically or by any one of the non-anatomical means (e.g. by osteotomy, etc.) implants are chosen.

For stable fractures, choice of an implant does not matter. For unstable fractures, sliding hip screw (DHS) is most suitable and the 135–150° angle side plates are most commonly used. Placement of the DHS screw in the neck should be either central or posteroinferior (Fig. 5.20).

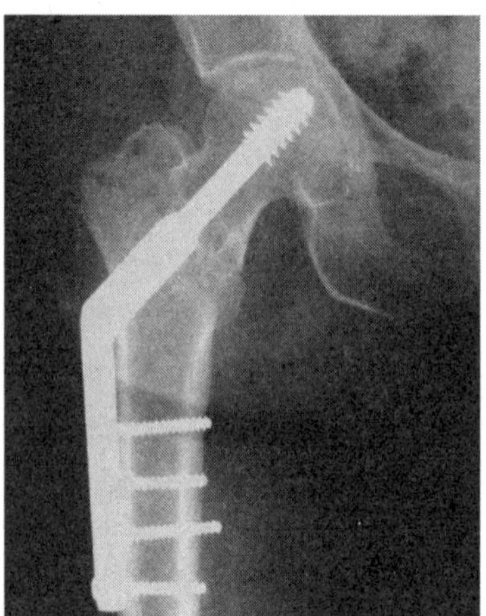

Fig. 5.20: Radiograph showing trochanteric fracture fixation with DHS

Dynamic hip screw (DHS) allows to secure fixation of the fracture and permits controlled impaction at the fracture site thereby reducing the risk of fixation failure seen in rigid nail-plate like SP nail, etc. (Fig. 5.21A). Proximal femoral Nailing (PFN) is being preferred over DHS in recent times (*see* box).

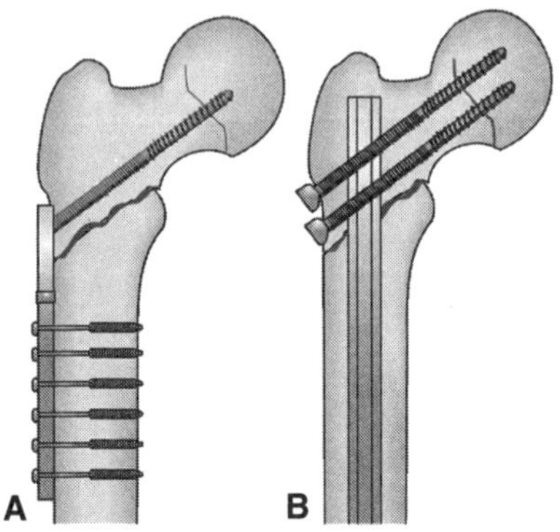

Figs 5.21A and B: Internal fixation methods for trochanteric fractures (A) DHS, (B) PFN

In intertrochanteric fracture, the success of fracture implant fixation depends upon:

- Degree of osteoporosis (Singh's index).
- Fracture pattern.
- Accurate reduction.
- Implant designs.
- Placement of the implant.

Vital facts

Treatment of Proximal Femoral Fractures

- Stable trochanteric fractures are fixed with DHS
- Unstable trochanteric fractures cannot be fixed with DHS as it cuts through due to comminution. Hence, the choice of implants in these situations is:
  a. Medoff plate or trochanteric stabilization plate (TSP, AO).
  b. *Condylocephalic nails:* These could be proximal femoral nails, Ender's nail or Gamma nail.
  c. 95° condylar blade plate or dynamic condylar screw.
  d. Proximal femoral nails (PFN) (Fig. 5.21B).

In comminuted unstable trochanteric fractures, IM nails are better suited to resist the deforming muscle forces. Hence, proximal femoral nailing is superior to DHS.

Advantages of PFN

- It can be inserted quickly
- Less blood loss
- Early ambulation
- Sliding and limb shortening is less
- It is more successful in reverse oblique fractures.

Features of PFN

- Standard length is 24 cm
- Long PFN is available in > 36 cm length (for low subtrochanteric fractures or two level fractures).
- *Proximal wide portion:* Here a long screw and hip-pin can pass through the head and neck.
- Distal part has a dynamic and static locking holes.

Problems with PFN

- Entry point has to be chosen carefully (preferably pyriformis fossa).
- Excessively curved femur is a central indication.
- Postoperative thigh pain is seen
- It cannot be used if fracture line extends into pyriformis fossa (Here DCS or condylar blade plate is better).

Now after having known the basic details of the injuries around the hip, let us try to know some of the common surgeries done around the hip.

BIBLIOGRAPHY

1. Allis OH. An enquiry into the difficulties encountered in the Reduction of Dislocations of the Hip, Philadelphia, Dornan printer, 1986.
2. Armstrong JR. Traumatic dislocation of the hip joint. Review of one hundred and one disorders. J Bone Joint Surg 1948;30 B:430-45.
3. Bigelow HJ. Luxation of the hip joint. Boston Med Surg J 1870;5: 1–3.
4. Birkett J. Description of a dislocation of the head of the femur complicated with its fractures. Trans, Med Chir Soc 1869;52:133.
5. BravEA. Traumatic dislocation of the hip. Army experience and results over a twelve-year period. J Bone Joint Surg 1962;44A: 1115–34.
6. Bromberg E, Weiss AB. Posterior fracture-dislocation of the hip. South Med J 1977;70:8–11.
7. Bucholz RW, Wheeless G. Irreducible posterior fracture dislocation of the hip. The role of the ilio-femoral ligament and the rectus femoris muscle. Clin Orthop 1982;167:118–22.
8. Butler JE. Pipkin type II fractures of the femoral head. J Bone Joint Surg 1981;63A:1292–96.
9. Catkins MS, Zycth G, Latta L, et al. Computed tomography evaluation of stability: Posterior fracture dislocation of the hip. Clin Orthop 1988;227:152–163.
10. Canale ST, Manugian AH. Irreducible traumatic dislocations of the hip. J Bone Joint Surg 1979;61A: 7–14.
11. Chakraborti S, Miller IM. Dislocation of the hip associated with fracture of the femoral head. Injury 1975;7:134–42.
12. Crock HV. An atlas of the arterial supply of the head and neck of the femur in man. Clin. Orthop 1980;152:17–27.
13. Delee JC. Dislocations and fracture dislocations of the hip, in: Rockwood CA. Green DP (Eds). Fractures and dislocations, 2 ed: Philadelphia JB. Lippincott, 1984;1287–1327.
14. DeLee JC, Evans JA, Thomas J. Anterior dislocation of the hip and associated femoral head fractures. J Bone Joint Surg 1984;62A:960–64.
15. Derian PS, Bibighaus AJ. Sciatic nerve entrapment by ectopic bone after posterior fracture-dislocation of the hip. South. Med J 1974;67:209–10.

16. Epstein HC. Traumatic dislocations of the hip. Clin Orthop 1973;92:116–42.
17. Epstein HC. Posterior fracture dislocations of the hip: Long-term follow-up. J Bone Joint Surg 1974;56A: 1103–27.
18. Epstein HC. Traumatic anterior dislocations of the hip. Management and Results. An analysis of fifty-five cases. J Bone Joint Surg 1972;54A:1561–62.
19. Epstein HC, Wiss DA, Coze L. Posterior fracture dislocations of the hip with fractures of the femoral head. Clin Orthop 1985;201:0–17.
20. Funsten RV, Kinser P, Frankel CJ. Dashboard dislocations of the hip. A report of twenty cases of traumatic dislocations. J Bone Joint Surg 1938;20:124–32.
21. Garrett JC, Epstein HC, Harris WH, et al. Treatment of unreduced traumatic posterior dislocations of the hip. J Bone Joint Surg 1979;61A: 2–6.
22. Hardinge K. The direct lateral approach to the hip. J Bone Joint Surg 1982;64B:17–19.
23. Hougard K, Lindenquest S, Nielsen LB. Computerized tomography after posterior dislocation of the hip. J Bone Joint Surg 1987;69B: 556–57.
24. Judet R, Judet J, le Tournel E. Fractures of the acetabulum. Classification and surgical approaches for open reduction. J Bone Joint Surg 1964;46A:1615–46.
25. Pipkin G. Treatment of grade IV fracture dislocation of the hip. J Bone Joint Surg 1957;39A: 1027–42.

Section II

Injuries of Spine

6

Spinal Injuries

The spine is an assembly of 33 bones running from the skull to the pelvis (Fig. 6.1). It has been assigned the twin responsibility of carrying the load of the body and head, thanks to the two-legged posture human beings enjoy and the still more important responsibility of protecting the vital spinal cord.

The neck bones (Fig. 6.2) are called *cervical vertebrae*, bones of upper back and in line with the chest are called *thoracic vertebrae* and the bones of the lower back are called *lumbar vertebrae*. Each vertebra rests on the vertebra above and below. At these points, they articulate with each other through the *facet* joint, which keeps all the vertebrae in their correct position and in alignment with each other. It has a spinal shock absorber called the *disk*, which separates each vertebra from the next.

Each vertebra has an *anterior body* and a *posterior neural arch* (Figs 6.3 and 6.4). The body has a tough outer cortex and a cancellous middle portion. It is supported in front and back by anterior longitudinal ligament and posterior longitudinal ligament respectively. The posterior neural arch consists of two pedicles, two transverse processes, a posterior spinous process and a pair of lamina, which together form the spinal canal along with the posterior surface of the body. In the canal lies the all-important spinal cord.

While ligamentum flavum binds the laminae together, the interspinous ligament binds the spinous processes, and the supraspinous ligament binds the tip of the spinous process. All the structures mentioned so far help in providing the much-needed stability.

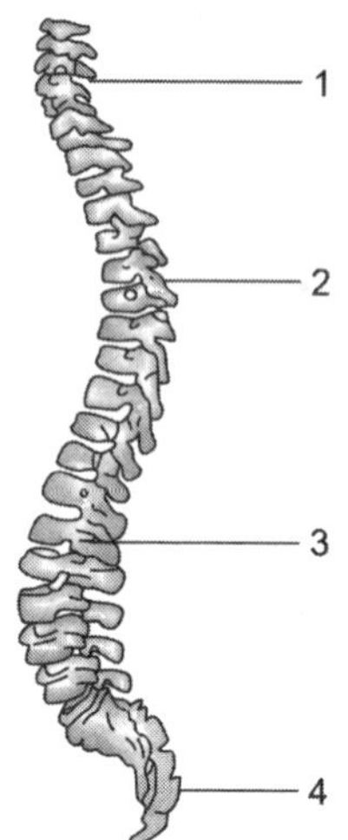

Fig. 6.1: Normal spinal curves: (1) Cervical lordosis, (2) Thoracic kyphosis, (3) Lumbar lordosis, and (4) Sacral kyphosis

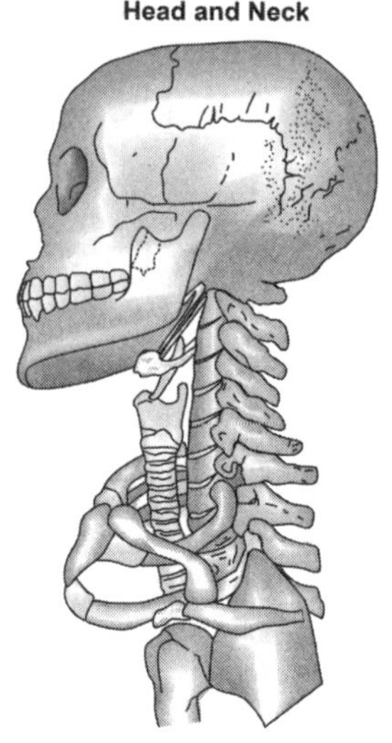

Fig. 6.2: Arrangement of the neck bones

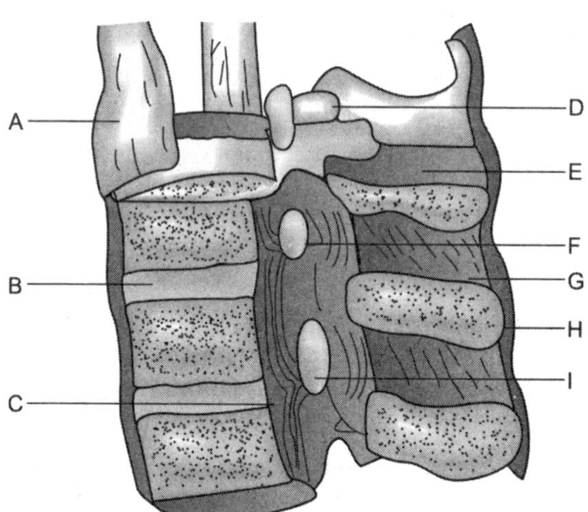

Fig. 6.3: Anatomy of spine: (A) Anterior longitudinal ligament, (B) Intervertebral disk, (C) Posterior longitudinal ligament, (D) Facet joint, (E) Interspinous ligament, (F) Ligamentum flavum, (G) Spinous process, (H) Supraspinous ligament, (I) Intervertebral foramen

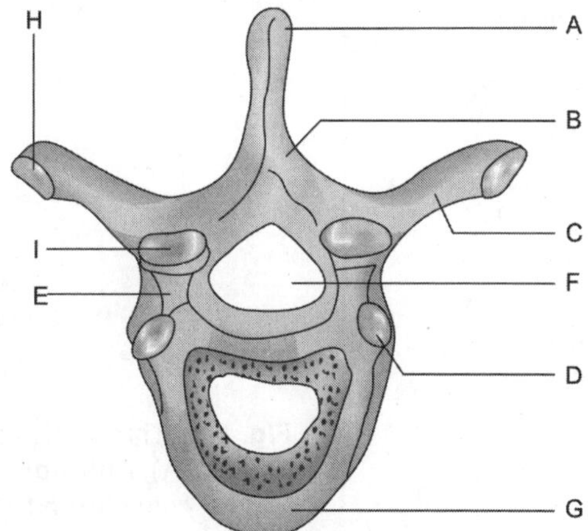

Fig. 6.4: Anatomy of a vertebra: (A) Spinous process, (B) Lamina, (C) Transverse process, (D) Superior articular facet, (E) Pedicle, (F) Spinal canal, (G) Body, (H) Transverse costal facet, (I) Inferior articular facet

When do we call spine as stable?

A spine, which after the initial injury refuses to be displaced further due to its intact posterior element, is called stable. Conversely, an unstable spine is one, which displaces further due to serious disruptions of the structures jeopardizing the spinal cord.

The *three-column concept* (Fig. 6.5) is the latest description of the spine stability. The *anterior column* consists of anterior half of the vertebral body, anterior part of the disk and anterior longitudinal ligament. The *middle column* consists of posterior half of the body and the disk, the posterior longitudinal ligament. The *posterior column* consists of the posterior vertebral arch consising of transverse process, spinous process and the accompanying ligaments. One column injury is stable, two column injury is unstable and three columns are invariably unstable. Unstable spine is a dangerous spine for it may injure the spinal cord.

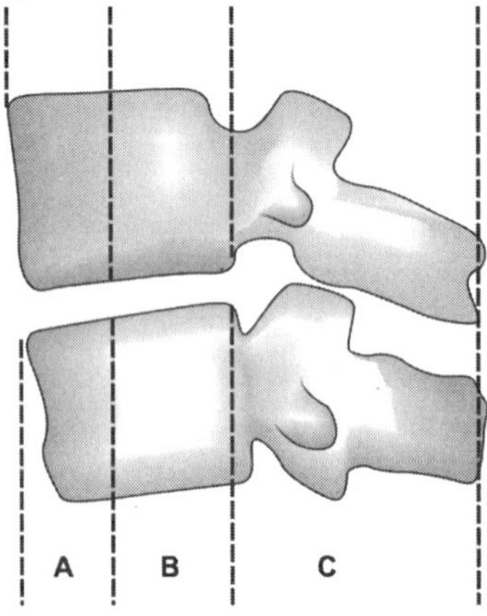

Fig. 6.5: Three-column concept of spine: (A) Anterior column, (B) Middle column, and (C) Posterior column

About spine

- It is the principal load bearing structure of the head and torso.
- Each portion of the spine has specific functions:
  Cervical spine provides head with limited mobility and protects proximal part of the spinal cord.
  Thoracic spine provides mobility to the upper torso and ribcage and protects the cord.
  Lumbar spine provides the lower torso, its mobility and protects the cord.
- Like the skull, which protects the brain, spinal column protects the cord.
- Spine should be flexible yet strong.
- Spinal cord injury could result in death, quadriplegia or paraplegia.

Disk facts

Functions of disk

- A disk has in the center nucleus pulposus and annulus fibrosus at the periphery.
- Binds vertebra together.
- Allows motion.
- Absorbs shock.
- Distributes load between the segments.
- Contributes to lordosis.
- Comprises approximately 25 percent of the total length of the spinal column.

Incidence of Spine Injuries

- About 1 million/year in the USA alone.
- Male : Female = 4 : 1.
- Injury is common at the cervicothoracic and thoracolumbar regions.
- Modes of injury
  - RTA—45 percent.
  - Falls—20 percent.
  - Sports injuries (diving)—15 percent.
  - Acts of violence—15 percent.

INJURIES OF THE CERVICAL SPINE

Injuries of the cervical spine are dangerous; and if associated with neurological damage, the results can be devastating. Though diagnostic and treatment methods have vastly improved over years, still injuries of the cervical spine pose the greatest challenge to the skill and acumen of orthopedic and neurosurgeons.

Jefferson pointed out two areas commonly involved in cervical spine injuries, C1-2 and C5-7. According to Meyer, C2 and C5 are commonly involved. Neurological damage is seen in 40 percent of cases. In 10 percent of cases, radiographs are normal.

Causes

Fall from height: It is the most common cause in developing countries.

Diving injuries: Diving into water with insufficient depth or in an inebriated condition.

Road traffic accidents (RTAs): Common cause in developed countries, e.g. whiplash injury (Fig. 6.6).

Gunshot injuries, etc. These injure the cervical spine and the cord directly.

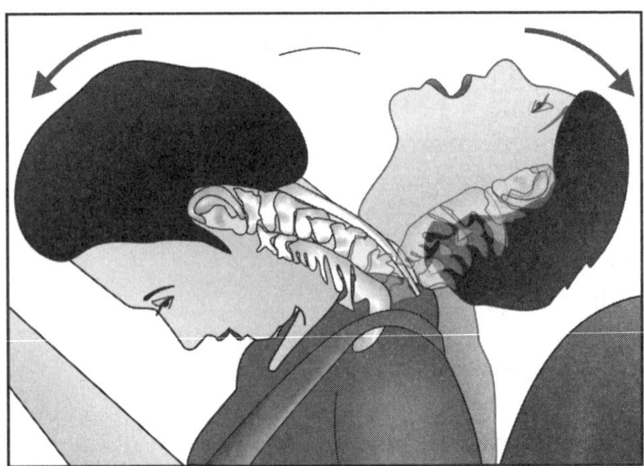

Fig. 6.6: Whiplash injury: Due to sudden deceleration, forceful hyperextension is followed by flexion of the neck

Mechanism of Injury (Figs 6.7A to D)

Pure flexion force: For example, compression fracture of vertebral body, e.g. fall from height.

Flexion rotation force: For example, fall on one side of the shoulder, disruption of facet capsule is seen.

Axial compression: For example, fall of an object on the head results in load compression, e.g. explosive comminuted fracture of C_5 body.

Extension force: For example, avulsion fracture of superior margin of vertebral body, e.g. whiplash injury.

Lateral flexion: For example, fracture pedicle, fracture transverse process and facet joints, etc.

Direct injuries: For example, fracture spinous process and body. Due to assault, gunshot injury, etc.

Whiplash Injury
(Syn: Acceleration injury, cervical sprain syndrome, soft tissue neck injury)

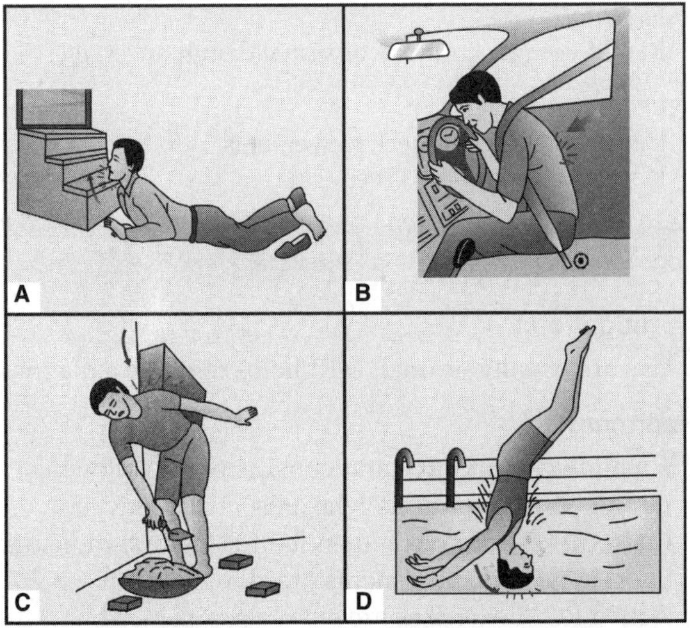

Figs 6.7A to D: Common mechanism of cervical spine injuries: (A) Hyperextension injury, (B) Flexion extension injury, (C) Flexion rotation injury, (D) Hyperflexion injury

Definition

It is an unconventional and inconsequential ligamentous injury of the cervical spine allegedly due to an extension injury following a rear-end collision in an RTA (Fig. 6.6).

Incidence

- It is seen in about 25 percent of rear-end collision of RTAs.
- Seventy percent of those affected are women.
- It is common in the 3rd or 4th decades.

Clinical Features

Symptoms

- Upper neck pain that becomes worse with movement.
- Occipital headache.

- Neck stiffness.
- Rarely vertigo, auditory or visual disturbances, etc.

Signs

- Decreased range of neck movements.
- Neck muscle spasm is seen.

Note: Symptoms appear within 48 hours of injury and 57 percent recover within three months. Final state is reached by one year.

Investigations

X-rays are usually normal. MRI helps to make a diagnosis.

Treatment

It is mainly conservative and consists of the following:

- *Drugs:* NSAIDs, muscle relaxants, etc. are given.
- *Collars:* These are recommended for the first three days.
- Short arc active movements are slowly begun.
- Active ROM exercises are slowly commenced.
- After the pain subsides, isometric strengthening exercises are slowly commenced.
- Other modalities take ultrasound, traction, manipulation, massage, etc. also helps.

Allen's Classification of Cervical Spine Fractures (Figs 6.8A to D)

Compressive flexion (5 stages): Ranges from blunting of anterosuperior vertebral margin to posterior displacement into the spinal canal. It is usually a stable fracture but may become unstable if compression is more than 50 percent.

Vertical compression (3 stages): Ranges from fracture of superior or inferior endplate with centrum fracture of the vertebral body. Stable fracture if compression is less than 50 percent of the vertebral body.

Distractive flexion (4 stages): Ranges from failure of posterior ligamentous complex to full-width vertebral body displacement. This is an unstable fracture.

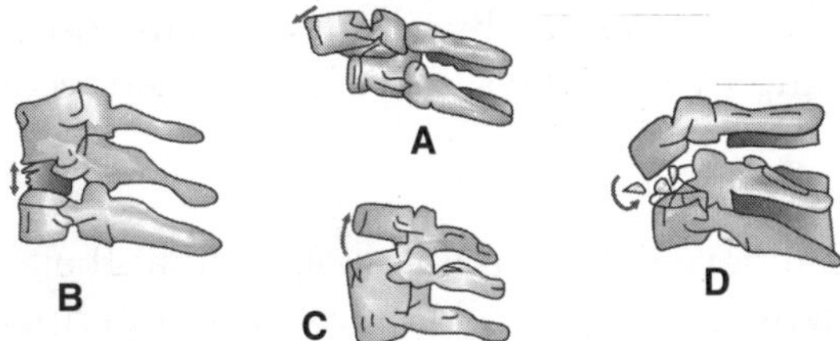

Figs 6.8A to D: Cervical spine injuries: (A) Distraction injury, (B) Compression injury, (C) Hyperextension injury, (D) Compression and distraction injury

Compression extension (5 stages): Ranges from unilateral vertebral arch fracture to bilateral vertebral arch fracture with full-vertebral body displacement anteriorly. It is unstable.

Distractive extension: Ranges from failure of anterior ligament complex to posterior ligament complex. This is also an unstable fracture.

Lateral flexion: Ranges from asymmetric compression and ipsilateral vertebral arch to fracture without displacement and with displacement. May become unstable.

Note: All unstable cervical spine fractures have a high incidence of neurological damage.

Clinical Features

The patient usually gives history of trauma following which there will be pain, swelling and inability to move the neck. There will be tenderness over the involved spinous process and there could be a palpable gap. There may be signs of neurological involvement. Determine the level of cord injury by examining the affected spine (see box). The injuries to the spinal cord at the cervical region can manifest in the following ways.

Concussion

This is a state of spinal shock and there will be sensory loss, flaccid paralysis, visceral paralysis, reflexes are in abeyance and anal reflex is absent. By 8 hours, concussion is known to regress; and by 8–10 days, there is complete recovery.

Nerve Root Involvement

Individual nerve roots could be affected at their respective intervertebral foramen. All the features of peripheral nerve injury with LMN type of lesion are seen. The myotome and the dermatome should be assessed to know the root involvement (Figs 6.9 to 6.16 and Table 6.1).

Cord involvement could be:
Complete: This leads to quadriplegia or quadriparesis.
Incomplete: Here the central cord, lateral cord, anterior or posterior cord could be involved (Table 6.2).

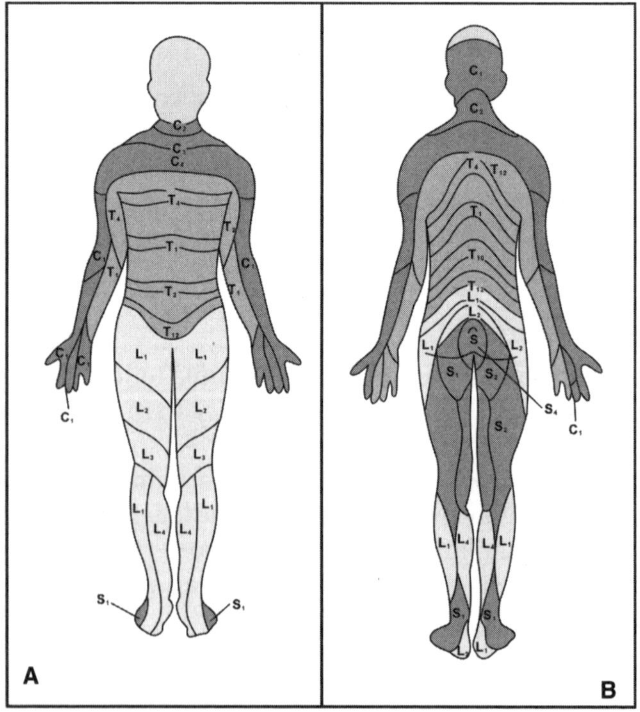

Figs 6.9A and B: Dermatomal levels: (A) Anterior, and (B) Posterior

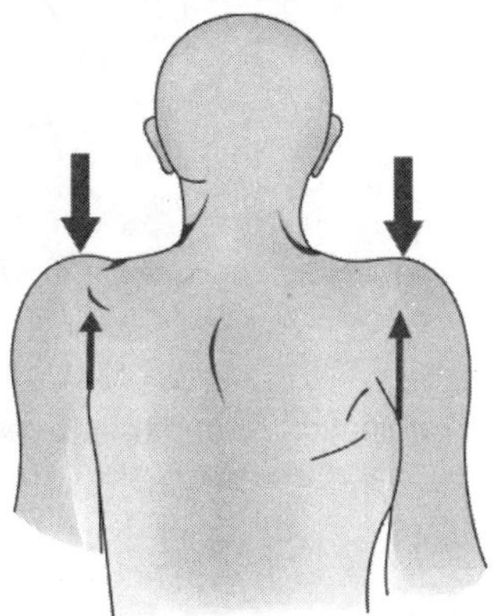

Fig. 6.10: Examination of C3-C4 (Trapezius muscle)

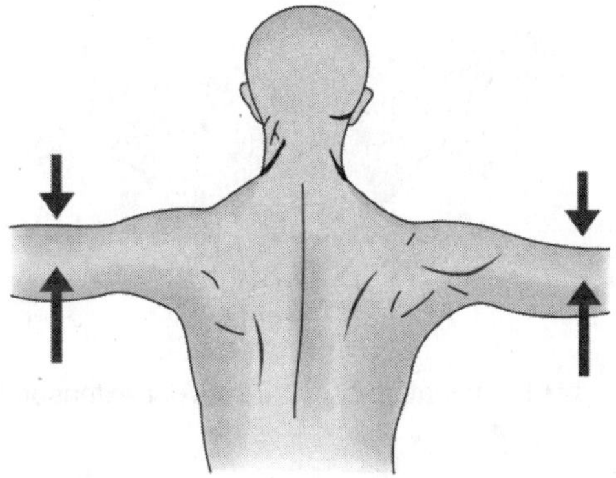

Fig. 6.11: Examination of C5–C6 roots (Deltoid muscle)

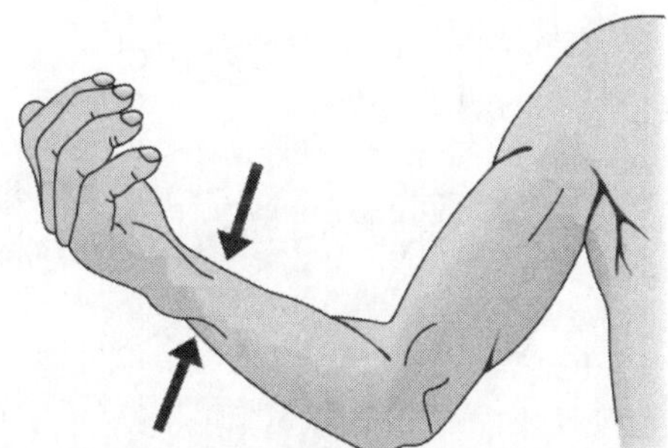

Fig. 6.12: Examination of C5–C6 roots (Biceps muscle)

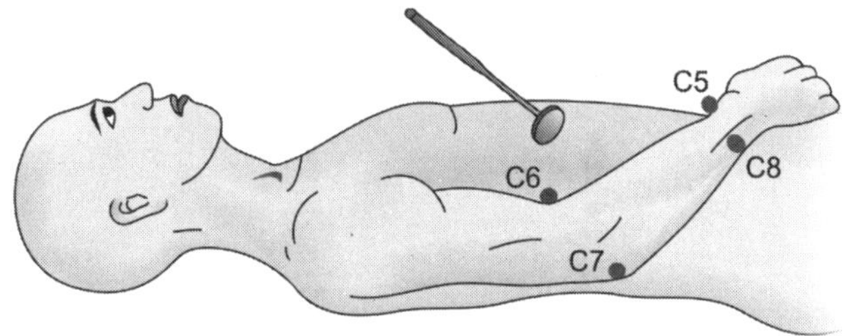

Fig. 6.13: Examination of upper limb reflexes

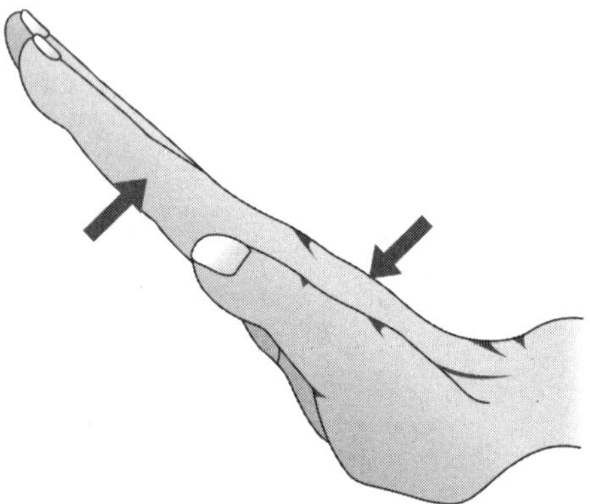

Fig. 6.14: Examination of C7-C8 (Wrist extensors)

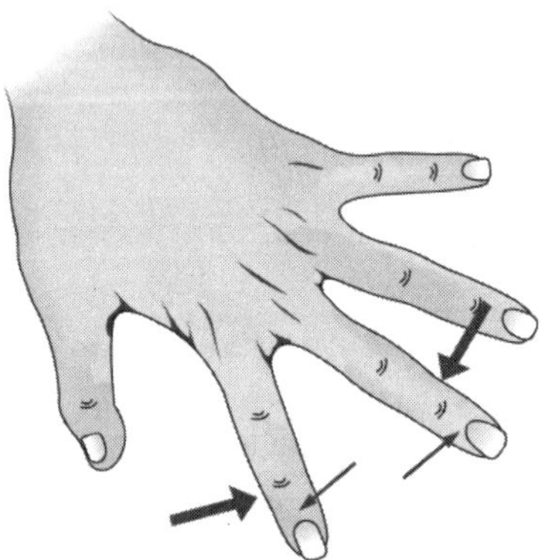

Fig. 6.15: Examination of C8-T1 (Dorsal interosseous muscle)

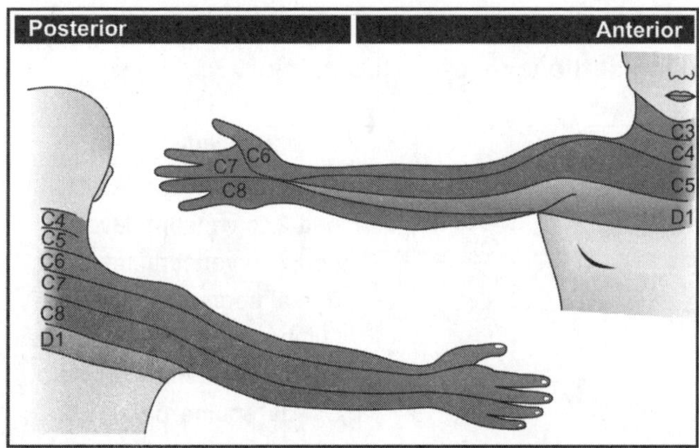

Fig. 6.16: Dermatomal pattern of cervical nerve roots

Table 6.1: Root involvement: quick facts

Roots	*Sensory system*	*Motor system*
C2	Sensation decreased over back of the scalp	C2-C4 root involvement survival of patient is rare
C3	↓sensation over anterior aspect of the neck	-do-
C4	↓sensation over lateral aspect of neck and inferiorly over clavicles down to the rib space	-do-
C5	↓sensation over the lateral deltoid	↓voluntary activity of deltoid and biceps
C6	↓sensation over the radial aspect of the forearm, thumb, index and middle finger	↓ECRL, ECRB activity
C7	↓sensation over the ulnar border of ring and small fingers	↓triceps, finger extensors, pronator teres, and FCR activity
C8	↓sensation over ulnar border of hand and forearm	↓FDS or profundus activity
T1	↓sensation over the medial aspect of the upper arm	
T2	↓over the anterior chest wall above the nipple	Intrinsic function of the hand is intact

Note: FCR—flexor carpi radialis, ECRL—extensor carpi radialis longus, ECRB—extensor carpi radialis brevis, FDS—flexor digitorum superficialis

Do you know how to find out the level of cord injury by looking at the level of vertebral injury?

Bone segment	*Cord segment*
C_1 to C_7	Add 1 to vertebral level
T_1 to T_4	Add 2 to vertebral level
T_4 to T_{10}	Add 3 to vertebral level
T_{10}	Dorsal segments complete
T_{12}	Lumbar segments complete
L_1	Sacral segments complete
Below L_1	Cauda equina paralysis

Table 6.2: Cervical spinal cord injury

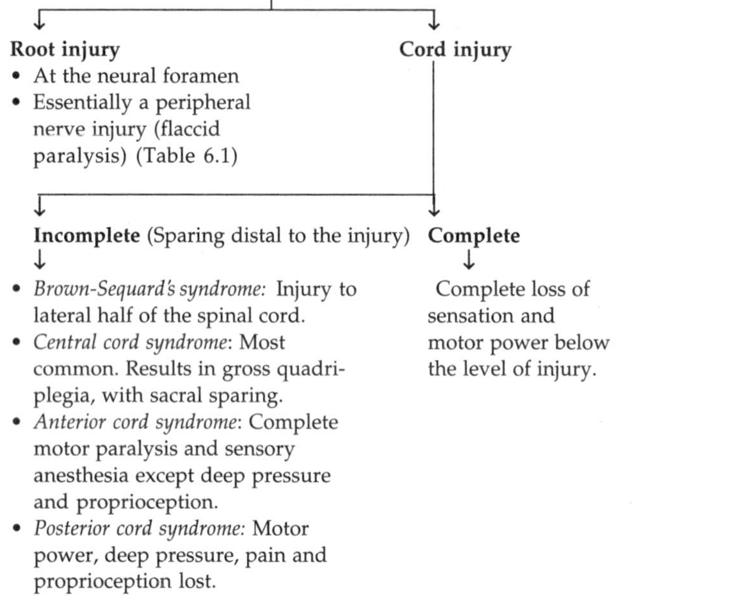

Vital Steps

- The lowermost functioning muscle is documented and a functional level is established.

- Next the sacrally innervated skin is examined. Perianal, anal, scrotal, labia, and plantar surface of the toes are examined.
- Perianal sensation may be the only sign to indicate an incomplete lesion.

Other Examinations

Rectal sensation: Loss of sensation around the anus.

Rectal motor: Sphincter contracts, over a gloved finger.

Bulbocavernosus reflex: Involves S_1, S_2 and S_3 nerve roots. Squeeze the glans penis, anal sphincter contracts around the gloved finger.

Initially, following the injury, the above reflexes are absent, indicating spinal shock. Usually, it returns within 24 hours. If not a presumptive diagnosis and determination of a root or cord lesion is made. A diagnosis of a complete or incomplete syndrome is documented.

Cord concussion

A state of "spinal shock", i.e. temporary electrical dysfunction.

Features

- Sensory loss.
- Flaccid paralysis.
- Visceral paralysis.
- Reflexes are in abeyance.
- Anal reflex lost (anal wink lost).

Usually

- Eight hours later concussion regresses.
- Seven to ten days later complete recovery. If the reflexes, do not return within 24 hours to 10 days a diagnosis of complete cord transection is made.

Investigations

Radiography: Lateral view is important (Fig. 6.17). If an adequate lateral radiography reveals no fracture or dislocation, then a complete radiographic examination including anteroposterior, open mouth and oblique projections are performed.

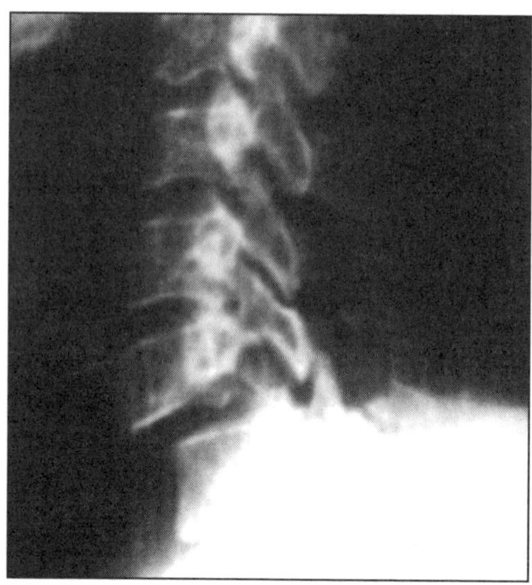

Fig. 6.17: Radiograph showing fracture dislocation of C6 over C7

Myelography is of value in incomplete lesion who fails to show progressive improvement.

CT scan makes an accurate diagnosis of hidden fracture. It is not helpful in assessing the soft tissue injury.

MRI evaluates cord injuries better. MRI is found to be very reliable and helpful in assessing the bony, soft tissue damages and injury to the cord very accurately.

General laboratory investigations: Like Hb percentage, blood group, bleeding time, clotting time, electrolyte status, etc. are done.

Treatment facts

Goals of treatment of cervical spine injury

- Realign the spine.
- Prevent further neurological damage.
- Aid neurological recovery.
- Obtain and maintain spinal stability.
- Aim at early functional recovery.

Treatment Methods

At the Accident Site

Resuscitation and transport is important. In a person lying still without using his neck after an RTA, a cervical spine injury is always suspected until proved otherwise.

The patient is transported with utmost care over a stretcher to the hospital. All unnecessary neck movements should be totally avoided. If the patient needs resuscitation, it has to be carried out with a lot of care.

At the Hospital

Nonoperative treatment: Most cases can be treated non-operatively by halo vest, four postcervical collars, Minerva jacket, cervical collars, etc. (Figs 6.18A to C).

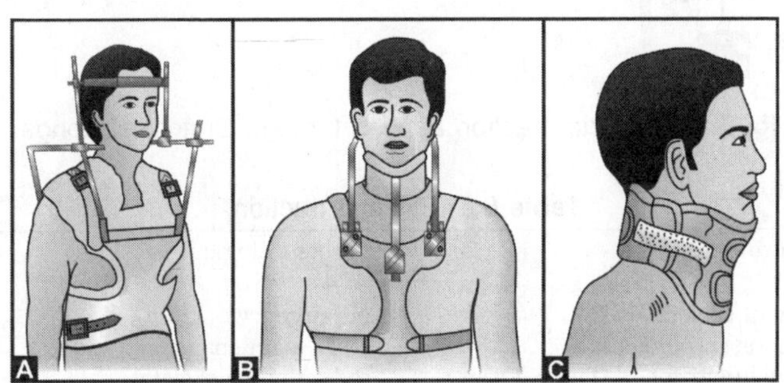

Figs 6.18A to C: Methods of cervical immobilization: (A) Halo-vest traction, (B) Four post cervical collar, (C) Cervical collar

Indications

- Stable cervical spine with no neurological injury. A rigid cervical brace or halo for 8–12 weeks is usually sufficient.
- Stable compression fracture of vertebral bodies and undisplaced fracture of laminae, lateral masses or spinous process.
- Unilateral facet dislocations reduced in traction may be immobilized in a halo vest for 8–12 weeks.

Skeletal traction: Reduction with traction is done for unstable fracture (Fig. 6.19). Urgency of reduction is based on neurological loss (Table 6.3). Traction is given for 3–6 weeks and once satisfactory reduction is achieved, the patient is mobilized with a collar, corset or jacket.

Halo Vest Immobilization: Many unstable cervical spine injuries can initially be managed by cervical traction through a halo ring. After obtaining the alignment of the cervical spine, halo vest may be completed.

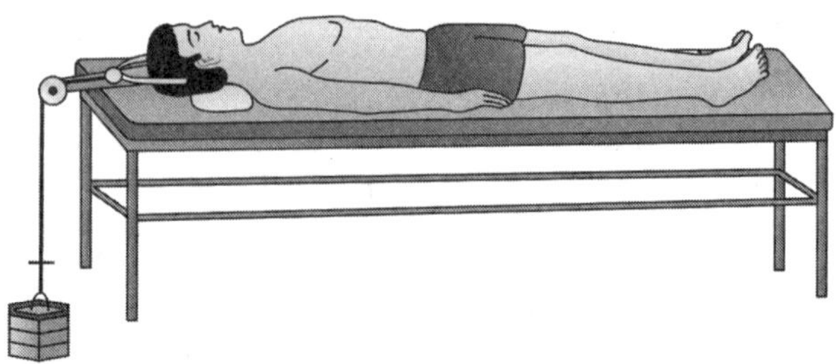

Fig. 6.19: Skeletal traction applied through Crutchfield tongs

Table 6.3: Skeletal traction

Neurologic loss	No neurologic loss
↓	↓
Urgent skeletal traction through Crutchfield tongs (Fig. 6.20) or Gardner-Wells tongs	No urgency Only maintenance of reduction of skeletal traction.
↓	
10 lbs weight for head, 5 lb weight for each vertebra to a maximum of 40 lb.	

If reduction is obtained, weight is ↓by 50 percent. If reduction is not obtained, open reduction is attempted.

Surgical Treatment

Indications: Unstable injuries with or without neurological damage require surgery.

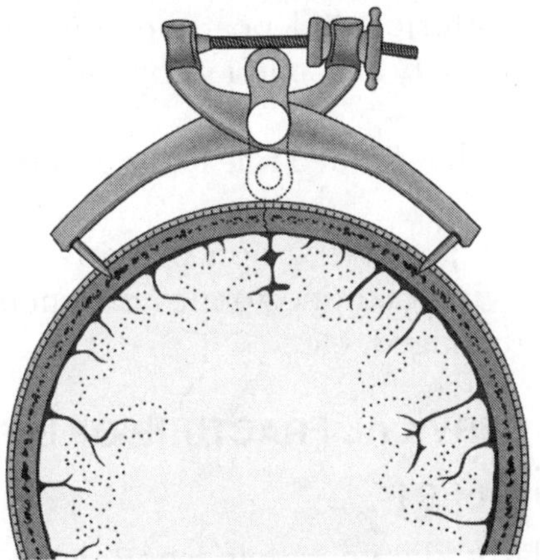

Fig. 6.20: Crutchfield tongs

Methods

- In most patients early open reduction and internal fixation (ORIF) is indicated to obtain stability. Cervical spine is stabilized through an anterior or posterior approach. Usually, a posterior approach is used with triple wire stabilization and fusion with iliac bone grafting. This allows rapid mobilization of the patient in a cervical orthosis.
- Anterior decompression consists of removal of the disk and is recommended when disk prolapse is present.
- Anterior cervical plating allows for immediate rigid fixation after decompression and bone grafting. The plates used are H-type or Caspar plates. Recently cervical spine locking plate (CSLP) and reflex anterior cervical plate are providing better fixation and faster rehabilitation.
- Posterior approach preferred for ligamentous instability. Posterior stabilization and rigid internal fixation is provided by systems like Roy-Camillie, Magerl and Seemann, etc. which have posterior plates and screws, hook plates, etc.
- Anterior approach and corpectomy (removal of the crushed body) for burst fracture with cord compression. After corpectomy, a bone graft or a cage fills up the gap.

- Combined anterior and posterior decompression for posterior instability and anterior compression of the neural elements.

Laminectomy has limited role in the treatment of cervical fracture.

Lateral mass screw fixation provides rigid internal fixation in previous laminectomies or when the spinous processes are damaged, etc.

INDIVIDUAL CERVICAL FRACTURE OF INTEREST

Burst Fracture of C1

This is popularly known as Jefferson fracture. It is due to axial loading over the top of the head. Here the patient usually presents with neck pain without neurological deficit. This can be radiologically diagnosed by open mouth odontoid view (Fig. 6.21).

Treatment

For stable fracture: Rigid cervicothoracic brace for three months with a Philadelphia cast.

For unstable fractures: Skeletal traction or halo traction for 3–6 weeks followed by application of halo vest.

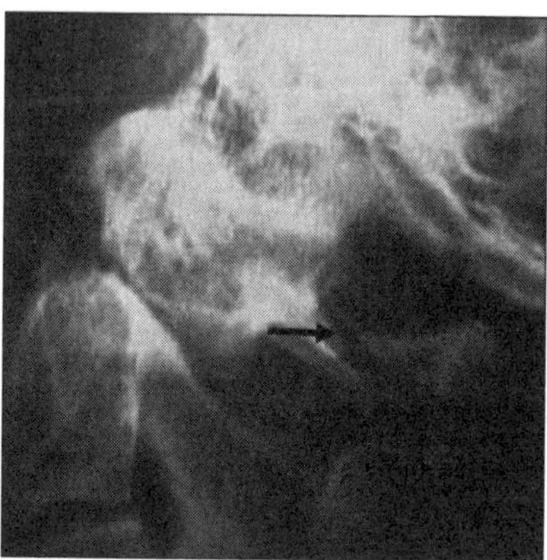

Fig. 6.21: Jefferson fracture

Rotary Subluxation of C1 or C2

Here the patient presents with torticollis and neck pain and is diagnosed radiologically. Treatment is usually by reduction and skull traction.

Odontoid Process Fracture

It is also called Dens fracture (Figs 6.22A to C).

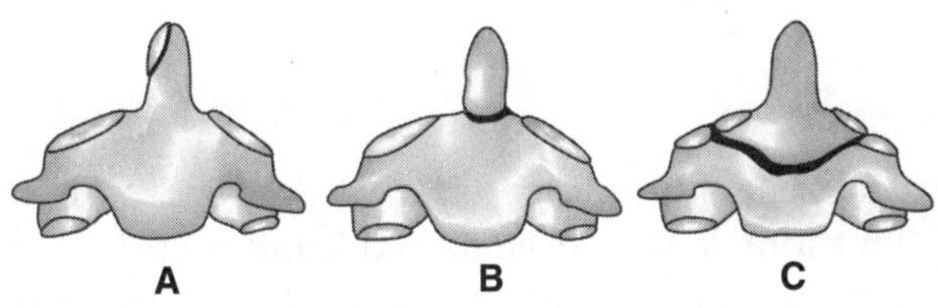

Figs 6.22A to C: Odontoid process fracture: (A) Type I, (B) Type II, and (C) Type III

Anderson and D'olonzo's Classification

Type I: Oblique fracture of the upper part of the odontoid process. It is uncommon and is treated by cervical cast.

Type II: Junction of odontoid process and body. Common with a nonunion rate of 36 percent. Requires surgical wiring and fusion.

Type III: Fracture is through the upper part body of the body of vertebra. Cancellous area hence fracture unites well with a halo cast.

Hangman's Fracture

It is a fracture through pedicle at pars-interarticularis of C_2 and is due to distraction extension force. There is no neurological deficit and the patient needs rigid cervical support usually through a Philadelphia collar immobilization.

7 Thoracic and Lumbosacral Spine Injuries

Introduction

Thoracolumbar spine is generally regarded as extending from 10th thoracic vertebrae to 2nd lumbar vertebrae and is the transitional area between the kyphotic upper thoracic spines to the lordotic lumbar spine. The general anatomy of the vertebral column is more or less the same as in other areas of spine. The three column concept has already been described. Anterior column is the load bearing structure and the posterior column functions as motion limiters as well as load bearing structures.

Mercifully, the thoracolumbar injuries spare the upper limbs and vital functions. Though a lesser challenge than cervical injury, nevertheless it poses problems, no less risky than the former.

Mechanism of Injury

- Fall from a height.
- RTA: Seat belt injury (chance fracture).
- Other causes like gunshot injuries, assault, etc.

McAfee's Classification—3-Column Classification (Figs 7.1A to D)

Wedge Compression

Isolated failure of anterior column due to forward flexion. No neurological deficit.

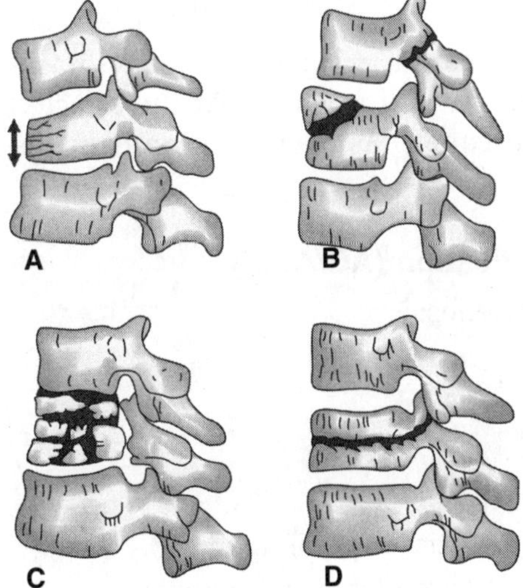

Figs 7.1A to D: Thoracolumbar fractures: (A) Wedge compression, (B) Stable burst fracture, (C) Unstable burst fracture, (D) Chance fracture

Stable Burst Fractures

Anterior and middle columns fail. No loss of integrity of posterior elements.

Unstable Burst Fractures

Anterior and middle column fail in compression. Posterior column fail in compression, lateral flexion or rotation. Post-traumatic kyphosis and neural symptoms are present.

Chance Fracture (Seatbelt injury)

It is seen in people who wear a lap belt without a shoulder harness. Horizontal avulsion fracture of vertebral bodies caused by flexion about an axis anterior to the anterior longitudinal ligament. A strong tensile force pulls entire vertebrae apart.

Flexion Distraction Injury

Flexion axis is posterior to the anterior longitudinal ligament. Anterior column fails in compression. Middle and posterior columns fail in tension. It is unstable because supraspinous, interspinous and ligamentum flavum fail.

Translational Injuries

Malalignment of neural canal, which has been totally disrupted. All three columns fail in shear. At the affected level, one part of sacral canal has been displaced in the transverse plane.

Modified Magerl Classification (AO/ASIF)

Type A: Compression varieties:

- Wedge.
- Split.
- Burst.

Type B: Distraction:

- Through posterior soft tissues (subluxation).
- Through the posterior arch (chance fracture).
- Through the anterior disk.

Type C: Multidirectional with translation:

- Anteroposterior dislocation.
- Lateral (lateral shear fracture).
- Rotational (rotational burst).

Clinical Features

The patient gives history of trauma due to RTA or fall from a height and complains of pain; posterior swelling, tenderness, palpable interspinous gap or a step may be felt. Neurological involvement may vary from paraplegia to individual nerve root involvement. Spinal shock is present for 24 hours during which all the reflexes are lost. Cauda equina paralysis is present if the lesion is below L_1. Exaggerated lumbar lordosis may be seen in old cases.

Investigations

Radiography of the affected spine this is the preliminary investigation and all three views (AP, lateral and oblique) are taken (Figs 7.2 and 7.3). Fracture of the vertebral body,

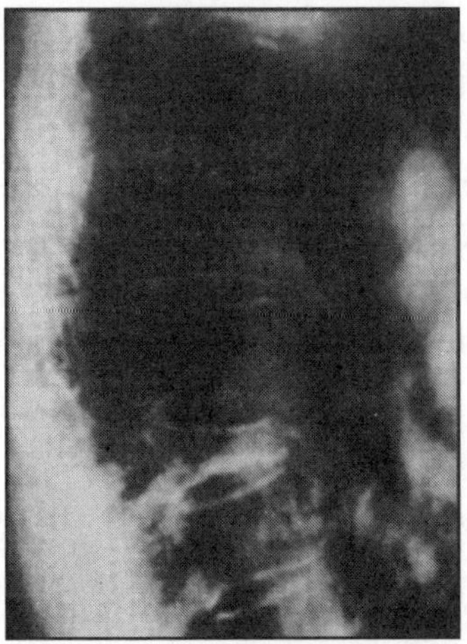

Fig. 7.2: Radiograph showing flexion compression fracture of T12 vertebra

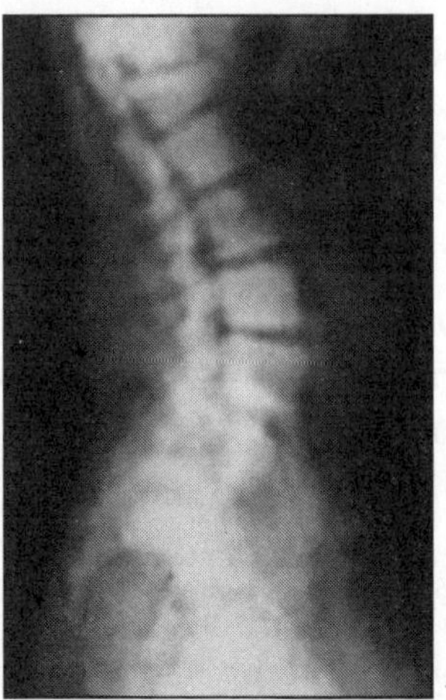

Fig. 7.3: Radiograph showing exaggerated lumbar lordosis due to L1 fracture

pedicles, lumbar transverse process, pedicles spinous process, etc. is looked for. Disk space and neural canal narrowing is looked for. With the advent of MRI and CT scan, the role of radiography appears to be diminishing in importance.

CT scan and MRI are found to be more useful than radiographs in evaluation of spinal trauma. While CT scan helps in studying the bony elements, MRI helps in the study of both bone and soft tissue elements. The damage to the cord is detected accurately and is now being considered as the "gold standard" in the investigation of spine injury.

Mystifying Facts: Radiological clues about an unstable spine

- Loss of vertebral height > 50 percent.
- Kyphosis > 30 percent.
- Spondylolisthesis > 3 mm.

Management

This is discussed under two heads.

Management at the site of accident: This consists of careful handling of the patient suspected to have spine injury. Consider all patients with spine injury to have neurological damage, shift them to the hospital with utmost care, and caution avoiding all unnecessary movements.

Definitive treatment at the hospital: The examination and the management measures practiced at the casuality are as follows:

Practice: Caution in handling the neck.

Examination: The general condition and other systems like CNS/CVS/RS/PA/GI tract, etc. Also, examine from head to toe, the presence of other fractures, head, chest injuries, blunt injury abdomen and pelvic fractures.

Evaluate: The spine injury by gentle careful clinical examination. This has to be supplemented by proper investigations like X-ray, CT-scan, MRI, etc.

Assess: Carefully assess the level and extent of neurological damage by examining the dermatome, myotome and reflexes.

Plan: After evaluating and assessing the damage, plan the line of treatment. The treatment options include nonoperative, traction and operative methods. Now let us carefully look into various treatment modalities.

This varies depending upon the nature of injury and the presence or absence of neurological damage (Flow chart 7.1):

- *For stable fracture without neurological deficit* Less than 30 percent anterior wedge, lateral, central compression fracture of the vertebral body is considered as stable fracture. In these injuries, there is no fracture of the posterior cortex of the vertebral body, and there is no disruption of the neural arch.

  Treatment: This is essentially conservative and consists of bed rest, NSAIDs and external spine supports like brace, corsets, etc. If the vertebral body compression is less than 30 percent, only corset is used; and if the compression is

Flow chart 7.1: Treatment plan for thoracolumbar injuries

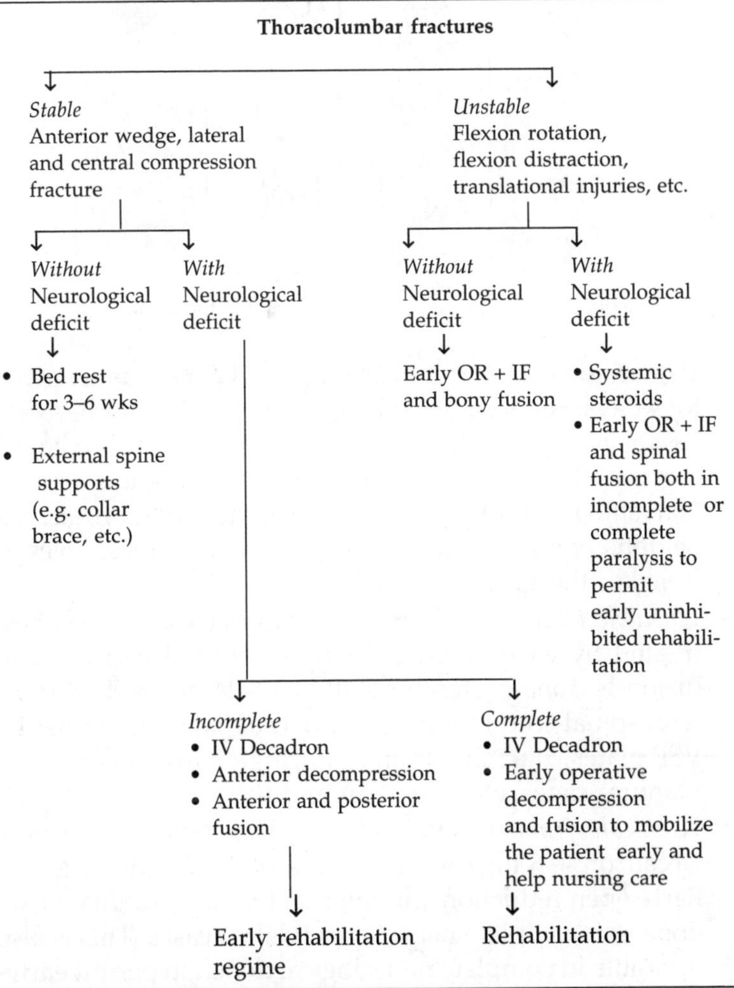

more than 30 percent but less than 50 percent, a plaster jacket along with a corset is preferred (Fig. 7.4).

- *For stable fracture with neural deficit:* It has to be first determined whether the neurological deficit is complete (loss of motor power, sensory loss and absent reflexes) or incomplete (only cord or only spinal nerve roots).

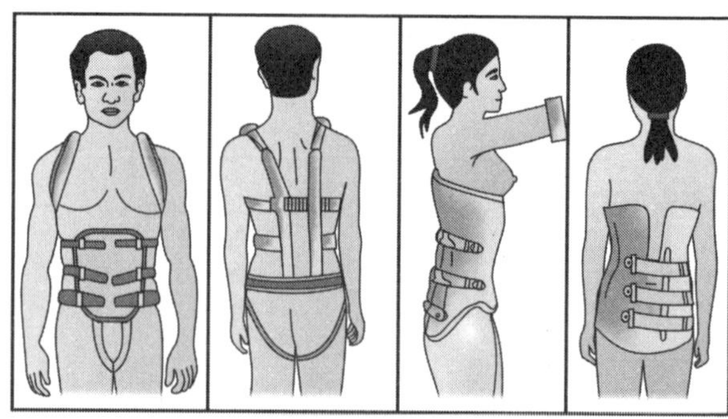

Fig. 7.4: Spinal braces for the treatment of stable thoracolumbar injuries

If neurological damage is incomplete, IV steroids are given for 4 days. Anterior decompression and anterior interbody fusion is done in the first stage, followed by posterior segmental spinal stabilization by either pedicle screws, Hart shill rectangle frame, Luque instrumentation, etc. can be done one week later. Laminectomy has fewer roles as it makes the spine less stable.

- *Unstable fracture without neurological deficit:* This is best treated by early open reduction, internal fixation and fusion is done preferably within 12–24 hours. It is done with spinal cord monitoring. Internal fixation is either by VSP plates, Hart shill frame, Harrington instrumentation, titanium cages, etc (Figs 7.5A and B).
- *Unstable fracture with neurological deficit:* Systemic Decadron 4–6 mg/every 6 hours IV for 3 days is given. Early open reduction and internal fixation and fusion are done in incomplete neurological deficit cases. This is also desirable in complete neurological deficit to permit early-uninhibited rehabilitation. Segmental spinal stabilization with Luque or Hart shill frame is recommended.

Fixation Choices

Posterior spinal instrumentation for lumbar fractures: Luque screw segmental spinal instrumentation is found to be very effective.

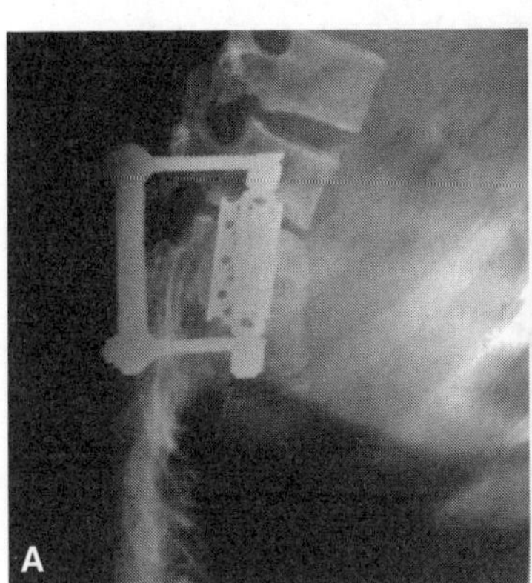

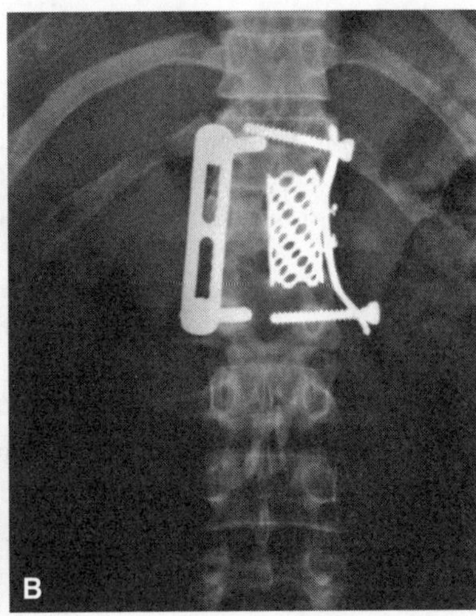

Figs 7.5A and B: (A) Radiograph showing posterior instrumentation (Lateral view) Fixation with cage, (B) AP view

Anterior spinal instrumentation for fractures from T_{10} to L_3 and used as a lateral vertebral body device. However, the procedure is more morbid and is associated with dangerous complications like vascular injury, etc. Anterior plate system can be used to manage the thoracolumbar burst fracture and strut grafts can easily be placed with this approach.

Anterior vertebral body excison: This is indicated in vertebral burst fractures of more than two weeks duration and who are not a candidate for posterior instrumentation. This is followed by strut grafting and internal fixation.

What is new in the treatment of vertebral compression fractures?

Vertebroplasty: This procedure consists of injecting bone cement under high pressure through large spinal needles into the acutely painful compressed and collapsed osteoporotic vertebral body. This is done mainly to relieve pain due to collapse of the body, strengthen it further to prevent future collapse and not done to restore the body height. Vertebroplasty is known to reduce pain in 70–90 percent of patients.

Balloon kyphoplasty: This is different from vertebroplasty in restoring the collapsed height of the compressed vertebral body by inflating a balloon inserted through small instruments through the pedicle. After restoring the height, a cavity is created, the balloon is deflated and withdrawn and the remaining cavity is filled with bone cement or graft under low pressure. This stabilizes the vertebra internally and relieves pain.

Both the above procedures are indicated in painful acute vertebral compression fractures in whom the medical management has failed.

What is new in the treatment of spine injuries?

Vertebroplasty: Injection of liquid cement into the vertebra through a key hole technique. This can be used along with the usual fixation methods to improve the stability.

8

Spinal Cord Injury

Spinal cord could be damaged due to injuries of spine extending from cervical vertebrae to the thoracolumbar junction. Below this, the cord ends and the cauda equina begin.

Incidence

- Spinal cord injuries are seen in 10–25 percent of cases of spinal column injuries.
- They are more common at the cervical level (40%) than the lumbar level (20%).

Pathology

The pathology may vary from extradural hemorrhage to cord concussion, laceration to cord crushing. Lesion has longitudinal, sagittal and coronal dimensions. Amount of neural damage has no relationship to radiographic appearance (Fig. 8.1).

Clinical Classification of Neurological Damage

- Complete paralysis.
- Sensory paralysis.
- Motor paralysis useless.
- Motor paralysis useful.
- Recovery.

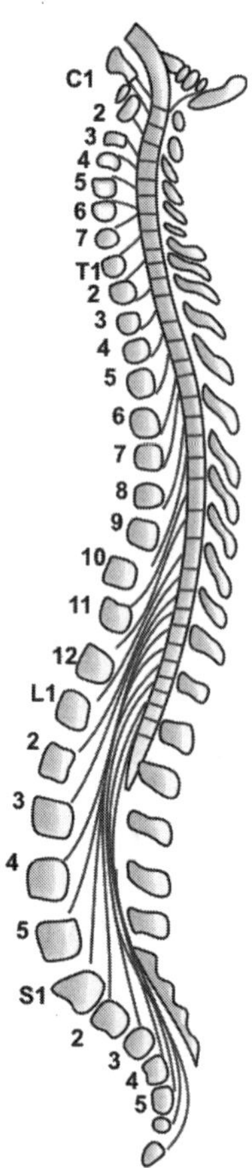

Fig. 8.1: Spinal cord ending at L1 cauda equina starting at this point

Injury at the cervical level: This has already been discussed and may vary from concussion, root injuries, incomplete and complete cord transection.

Injuries at the thoracic level: This could result in paraplegia.

Injuries at the thoracolumbar region: Due to injuries at the thoracolumbar junction, three things can occur:

- Complete cord division and nerves intact.

- Complete cord division and partial nerve division.
- Complete cord division and complete nerve division.

Injuries below L_1 causes cauda equina paralysis.

Clinical Assessment

General examination: This consists of examination of the head, chest, pelvis and other systems for incidence of injuries and recording the vital statistics.

Neurological examination: Examine the level of the vertebral injury and find out the level of the corresponding cord injury (see box). Now each muscle group and dermatome has to be checked. In cases of cervical cord injury, survival is impossible if the cord is injured above C_4 level due to paralysis of the diaphragm and respiratory muscles. In injuries below C_4 and above C_7, the level of lesion can easily be detected by examining the respective myotome, dermatome and reflexes. In cases of injury at the thoracolumbar junction, a mixed picture of both cord and root lesion may emerge and there could be an UMN and LMN feature in the lower limbs. Below the L_1, it is the nerve roots, which are damaged, and it is easy to identify the injured nerve root by a careful examination of myotome, dermatome and reflexes of the lower limb. Slightest voluntary movement and sensation below the level of cord lesion indicate cord continuity with better prognosis. If paralysis is complete even after 8 hours and if there is symmetrical returning of reflexes and priapism in male, it indicates an unfavorable prognosis.

Return of reflex activity (e.g. anal reflex, bulbocavernosus reflex and plantar response): Return of reflex activity below the lesion indicates that the spinal shock has passed off and remaining paralysis and anesthesia may be due to injury to the long tracts of cauda equina.

Total sensory and motor paralysis after 8 hours with return of reflex activity indicates that distal part of spinal cord has been separated from cerebral control.

Nerve wracking points: Remember the Neurological facts

- Cervical spine level as mentioned previously.
- Between T_1 and T_{10}: Paralysis of trunk and lower limb muscles.
- At T_{10}: Paraplegia and the corresponding cord damage is at L1.
- Between D_{11} and L_1: Paraplegia and here the lumbar and sacral sections of the spinal cord are damaged along with their nerve roots.
- Below L_1: No cord damage, only root damage leading to cauda equina paralysis.

So to arrive at the proper level of spinal and cord damage, remember this rule:

Do you know how to find out the level of cord injury by looking at the vertebral injury?

Bone segment	*Cord segment*
C_1 to C_7	Add 1 to vertebral level
T_1 to T_4	Add 2 to vertebral level
T_4 to T_{10}	Add 3 to vertebral level
T_{10}	Dorsal segments complete
T_{12}	Lumbar segments complete
L_1	Sacral segments complete
Below L_1	Cauda equina paralysis

Investigations

This consists of plain radiograph of the affected part and all three views—anteroposterior, lateral and oblique are done. MRI and CT scan are also done and their role has already been described.

Treatment

- First aid as already discussed.
- Management of vertebral fracture and dislocations as discussed in individual injuries.
- Rehabilitation programs in neurological injury following spinal fracture are as follows:

Paralyzed Bladder

Bladder injuries could be either UMN type or LMN type (Table 8.1).

Table 8.1: Characteristic features of UMN and LMN bladder injuries

Bladder	*Automatic*	*Autonomous*
Type	UMN	LMN
Level	Above S_2	S_2 and below
Reflex center of bladder	Takes over	Lost
Controlled by	Reflex center	Intrinsic plexus of bladder
Emptying by	Involuntary	Voluntary
Residual urine	Minimal	Large > 200–300 cc

Goal in either case is to attain an automatic reflex emptying of the bladder.

UMN Type (automatic bladder)

This is seen in injury above S_2 due to complete transection of the cord. Here the bladder is distended and there is no real sensation of vesical filling and the bladder is controlled by the reflex centers. There is automatic involuntary emptying and no residual urine is left.

LMN Type (autonomous bladder)

This occurs in injuries at or below S2. The bladder reflex center is destroyed. It now depends on the intrinsic plexus in the musculature of the bladder wall (detrusor ganglion). Here, emptying is to be done by manual pressure or by trained contraction of abdominal musculature. There is a large amount of residual urine in this condition.

Treatment: In either condition mentioned above, the treatment method aims at obtaining automatic reflex emptying. This is done as follows:

- Urinary retention catheter is placed in the bladder for 24–48 hours.
- After 48 hours, intermittent catheterization is started, to develop the automatic reflex emptying of the bladder.

- Persons with traumatic quadriplegia have a UMN bladder controlled by reflexes through conus medullaris.
- If intermittent catheterization is not available, bladder range of motion exercises are performed by clamping the catheter tube for 50 minutes and opening for 10 minutes every hour to allow the bladder to develop a reflex pattern of emptying.
- If reflex emptying with residual bladder urine volume of less than 100 cc does not occur within 6-9 months, urological procedures like external sphincterotomy or bladder neck resection is done to achieve a balanced bladder.
- Urinary diversion through ileal loops, etc. is not superior to reflex emptying of the bladder and hence is not recommended.

All possible attempts should be made to remove the catheter and have a catheter-free reflex emptying of the bladder.

Bedsore Management

Preventing Bedsores (Figs 8.2 and 8.3)

Nursing goals: Education of the patients and relatives.

- Only sure method of preventing pressure ulcers is strict nursing care and gradual shifting of responsibility of the skin care to the patient's family.
- Spinal beds, mattresses and pads are not reliable to prevent pressure sores.

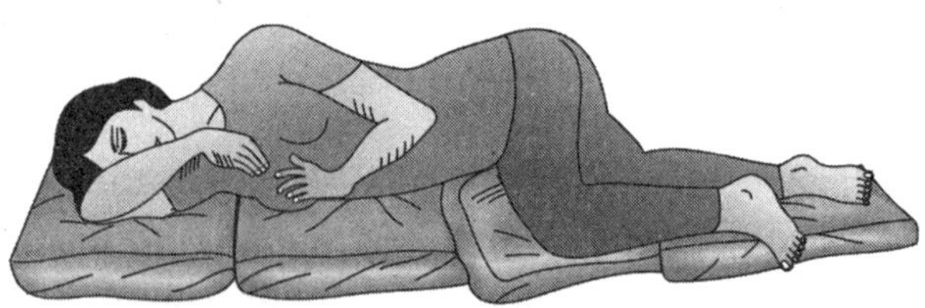

Fig. 8.2: Bed posture (side lying) to prevent formation of bedsores

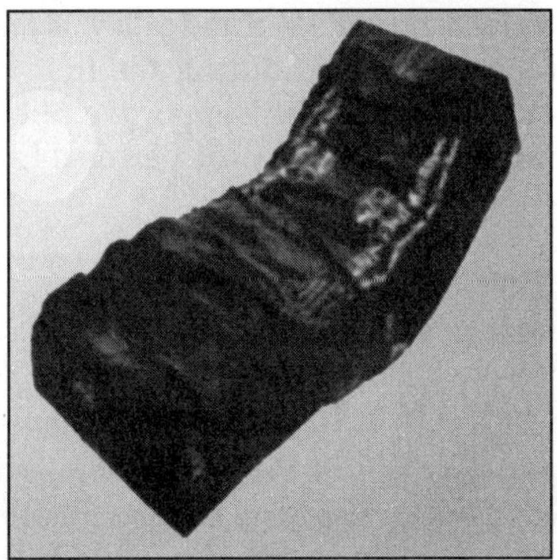

Fig. 8.3: Waterbed, a boon for prevention of bedsores

- Sleeping in prone position with a pillow bridging the bony prominences is the most reliable method of preventing bedsores.
- Using water bed also helps prevent bedsores.

Managing Bedsores

While prevention is the best mantra, the following measures are recommended once a bedsore develops:

- Keep the back dry.
- Apply a dry powder on the back.
- Turn the patient every 2 hours.
- Use water or air beds.
- Do periodic dressings taking all aseptic precautions.

Bowel Program

Reflex emptying of the bowel with suppository stimulation is the goal of bowel training: Every second or third day bowel reflex is stimulated by insertion of glycerin or Dulcolax suppository with digital stimulation. Enemas should not be given as this destroys the bowel reflex. Stool softeners and mild laxatives may be necessary.

Beds: A conventional hospital bed and pillow is preferred. Side-to-side rotating bed is used during the first week. Proper positioning of the patient with supportive pillows, frequent turning in the bed and care towards personal hygiene is very much needed.

Concept of Rotating Beds

- All spine injuries are placed on rotating beds in the causality.
- The bed rotates 40° on either side.
- Rotation stopped only for 2 hours in 8 hours.
- Safety straps and pads are applied firmly.
- Extremity exercises are permitted.
- Compression stockings to prevent thromboembolism.
- Spirometry is done every 2 hours.
- All investigations, MRI, X-ray, etc. can be carried out.
- The patient can be mobilized once the condition and the spine are stable.

Vital facts

Who require rotating bed treatment?

- Two to three column injury patients.
- Bony injuries without posterior ligamentous disruption.
- For individuals who are neurologically normal and improving.

Advantages

- The patient is comfortable.
- Nursing care becomes easy.
- Investigations, exercises, etc. can safely be done.

Family education: The family members of the victim are trained to take care of the victim's bowel, back, bladder and bed. They are also encouraged to give all the necessary moral support, which is so essentially required to rehabilitate the patient back to normalcy.

Physical therapy: This consists of putting joints through all the range of movements by passive stretching and exercises. Parallel bar walking, walking with the help of walkers or crutches is encouraged (Fig. 8.4). Wheel chair transfer activities are encouraged for injuries from C_6 level onwards.

Occupational therapy: If possible, the patient is allowed to return to his original work with minor adjustments if necessary. Nevertheless, if the patient, however, is unable to return to his

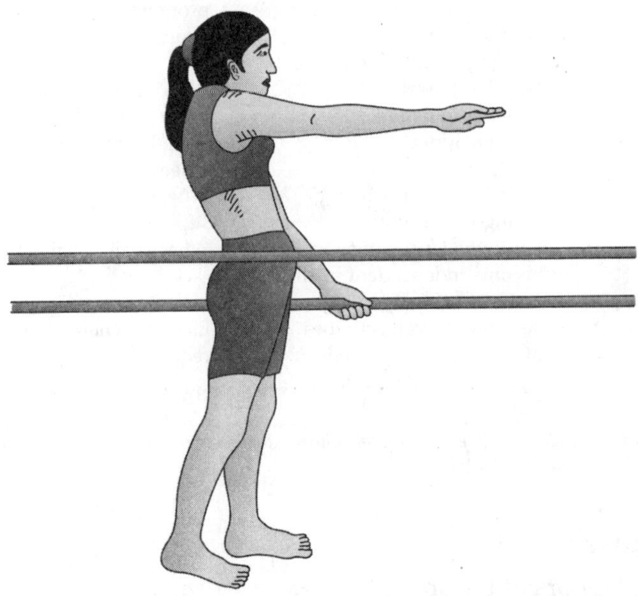

Fig. 8.4: A paraplegic patient learning to balance and walk within a parallel bar

original work, an alternative employment depending upon his present status of health is suggested.

Social therapy: The attitude of the people towards these patients should not be of sympathy, but of support and encouragement. The right attitude of the society towards these unfortunate victims will go a long way in rehabilitating them back to normal.

Table 8.2 shows various rehabilitative measures to be taken in patients with paraplegia.

CAUDA EQUINA SYNDROME

Cauda equina syndrome is seen in injuries below the level of first lumbar vertebra. It is essentially injury to the nerve roots below L_1.

Table 8.2: Rehabilitative measures for neurological injury

Level	*Disabilities*	*Measures*
$S_{2,4}$	Only bowel and bladder injured	Bladder and bowel program
L_4-S_1	Bladder, bowel and prolonged sitting impaired	Short leg braces
$L_{1,2,3}$	Bladder, bowel and walking impaired	Walking with long leg brace
T_7-$_{12}$	UMN bladder	Long leg brace and wheelchair
T_2-T_6	Bowel, bladder, walking, sitting impaired	Wheelchair is a must
C_7-T_1	Up to the level patient can become independent in all activities of daily living	Wheelchair is a must
C_5	Assistance to all activities of daily living required	Electrical chair is required
Above C_5	Total dependence + impaired Breathing	

This table shows the level of spinal injuries, their corresponding disabilities and the measures to be followed.

Causes

- Tumors of the spine.
- Pott's disease.
- Protrusion of disk—large midline disk prolapse at 4–5.
- Fracture dislocation of the thoracolumbar spine.

Clinical Features

Symptoms

The patient complains of back pain, perineal pain, difficulty in micturition, impotence in male, etc.

Sensory signs: The most salient feature of a cauda equina lesion is an area of *saddle-shaped hyperesthesia and later anesthesia* (involving buttocks, anus and perineum) (Fig. 8.5).

Motor signs: Flaccid paralysis below the knee.

Reflexes: Ankle jerk is lost and the knee jerk is increased due to the weakness of the opposing hamstrings.

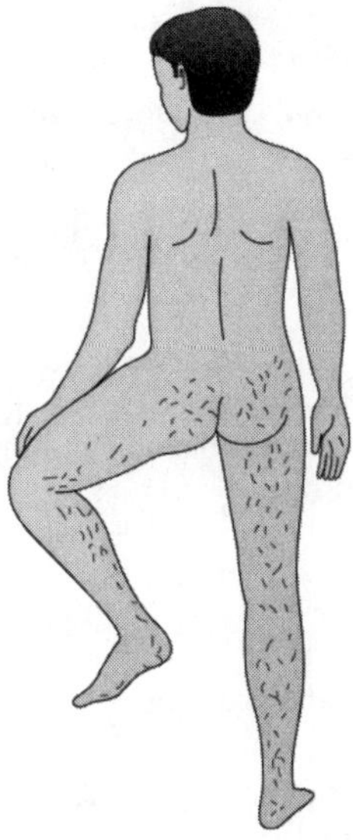

Fig. 8.5: Cauda equina lesion

Bladder symptoms: Common problems are retention of urine with overflow. Even after a severe cauda equina, lesion reflex micturition is established later, reflex being mediated through the vesical plexus.

Anal sphincter relaxation: leading to incontinence of the bowels.

Investigations

Plain X-ray, CT scan, MRI of the affected part is recommended.

Treatment

Prompt surgical intervention is the treatment of choice. This consists of operative stabilization of the fractures, bowel, back and bladder care and other rehabilitating measures have already been described above.

Prognosis in Spinal Cord Injuries

Ten-year survival rate in spinal cord injury is 86 percent.

Vital facts

Do you know the chief causes of death in spinal cord injuries? Well it is:

- Pneumonia
- Suicides

Interesting facts

Do you know what 'SCIWORA' is?
Well it is spinal cord injury without radiological abnormality. It is more common in children < 10 years.

BIBLIOGRAPHY

1. Crutchfield WG. Fracture dislocations of cervical spine. Am J Surg 1937;38:592.
2. Crutchfield WG. Skeletal traction in the treatment of injuries to the cervical spine. JAMA 1954;155:29.
3. Davis L. Treatment of spinal cord injuries. Arch Surg 1954;69:488.
4. Dickson JH, Harrington PR, Erwin WD. Harrington instrumentation in the fractured, unstable thoracic and lumbar spine. Texas Med 1973;69–91.
5. Holds worth FW. Traumatic paraplegia. In Platt H (Ed), Modern Trends in Orthopedics (2nd series), New York: Paul B, Hoeber, Inc 1956.
6. Holds worth FW. Fractures, dislocations, and fracture-dislocations of the spine. J Bone Joint Surg 1970;52-A:1534.
7. Jefferson G. Fracture of the atlas vertebra: Report of four cases and a review of those previously recorded. Br J Surg 1920;7:407.
8. Kelly RP, Whitesides TE (Jr). Treatment of lumbodorsal fracture dislocations. Am Surg 1968;167:705?
9. Maffee PC, Youn HA, Lasada NA. The unstable burst fracture. Spine 1982;7:365.
10. Watson-Jones R. Fractures and joint injuries (4th edn), Baltimore: Williams and Wilkins Co. 1952;1, 1955, 2.

9

Peripheral Nerve Injury

ULNAR NERVE INJURY

Course of the ulnar nerves and their supply is shown in Fig. 9.1.

Causes of Ulnar Nerve Injury

General Causes

These are due to diseases like leprosy, etc.

Local Causes

These are more important and could be in the following areas:

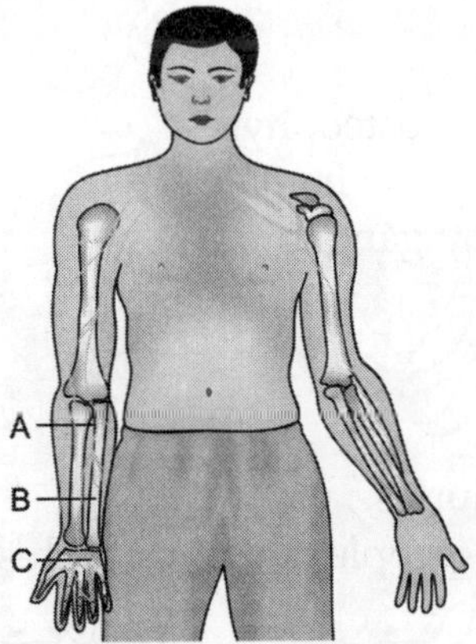

Fig. 9.1: Course of the median and ulnar nerves and their supply: (A) Flexor carpi ulnaris, (B) Flexor digitorum profundus, (C) Intrinsic muscles of the hand

Causes in the axilla
- Crutch pressure.
- Aneurysm of the axillary vessels.

Causes in the arm
- Fracture shaft of humerus.
- Gunshot and penetrating injuries.

Causes at the elbow
- Compression by the accessory muscle (anserina epitrochlearis).
- Fracture lateral epicondyle of humerus.
- Repeated occupational strains.
- Recurrent subluxation of the nerve.
- Compression by the osteophytes as in rheumatoid and osteoarthritis.
- Cubitus valgus deformity due to various causes results in repeated friction of the nerve giving rise to tardy (late) ulnar nerve palsy.

Causes in the forearm
- Fracture both bones forearm.
- Incised wounds, gunshot wounds and penetrating injuries of the forearm.

Causes at the wrist
- Compression by osteophytes.
- Fracture hook of the hamate.
- Compression by ganglion.
- Wrist injuries.

Causes in the hand
- Blunt trauma.
- Penetrating injuries.
- Occupational—people operating high-speed drills in rock mining, etc.
- Associated ulnar artery aneurysm.

Ulnar nerve injuries give rise to *claw hand* deformity either true type or ulnar claw hand.

CLAW HAND

It is a deformity with hyperextension of the metacarpophalangeal joints and flexion of the interphalangeal joints of the fingers.

Types and Causes

Two varieties are described: One is a true claw hand involving both median and ulnar nerves and the second an ulnar claw hand or claw-like hand due to ulnar nerve injury.

Problems of claw hand

- Hyperextension of MP joints (not the only primary or most disabling deformity).
- Grasp decreased by 50 percent due to loss of power of flexion at MP joints.
- Pinch decreased due to loss of stabilizing effect from the intrinsics.
- Roll up maneuver lost.
  Many surgical procedures are devised to block hyperextension of MP joints as it is still considered as the primary deformity.

Note: MP—Metacarpophalangeal, IP—Interphalangeal.

Clinical Features

These include the classical deformity, loss of sensation along the ulnar nerve distribution and wasting of the hypothenar muscles, intrinsic muscles of the hand leading to hollow intermetacarpal spaces on the dorsum of the hand (Figs 9.2A to C).

A test for loss of sensation along the distribution of the ulnar nerve in the hand and fingers is carried out. However, the clinical features vary depending upon the level of lesion.

Clinical Tests

For Ulnar Nerve Injury

Froment's sign: This is a reliable clinical test for ulnar nerve injury (Fig. 9.3). Three muscles (first palmar interossei, adductor pollicis and flexor pollicis longus) are required to

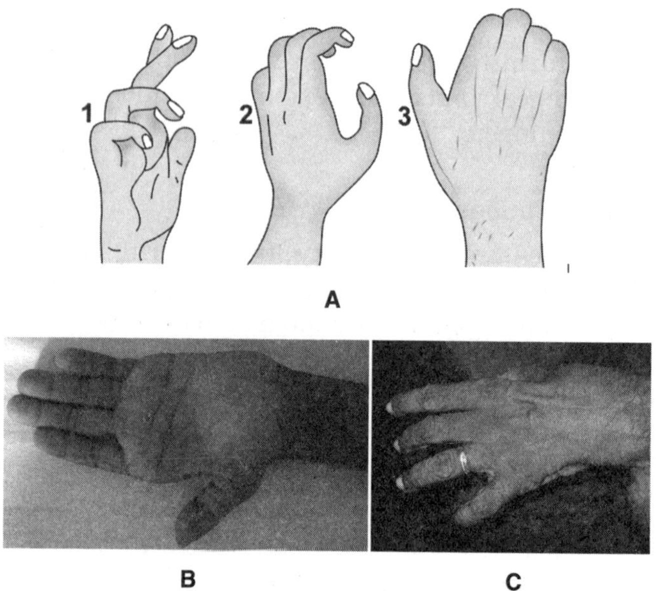

Figs 9.2A to C: (A) (1) Ulnar clawing, (2) Total clawing, and (3) Wasting of intermetacarpal spaces, (B) Hypethenar muscle wasting (clinical photo), (C) Intermetacarpal spaces (clinical photo)

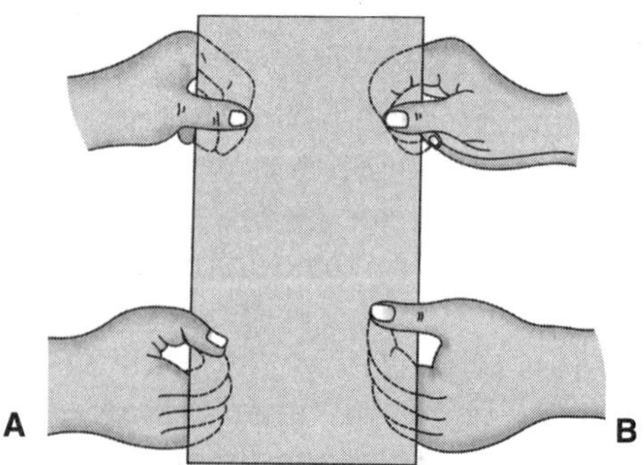

Figs 9.3A and B: Froment's sign: (A) Normal, (B) Ulnar nerve injury

hold a book between the thumb and other fingers. In ulnar nerve injury, the first two muscles are paralyzed and now to hold the book, the patient has to depend only on flexor pollicis longus, which flexes the thumb prominently. This is the positive Froment's sign.

Card test: Inability to hold a card or paper in between fingers due to loss of adduction by the palmar interossei (Fig. 9.4).

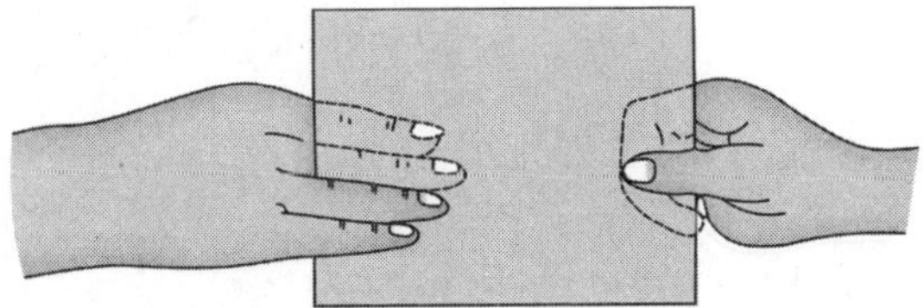

Fig. 9.4: Card test

Egawa test: With palm flat on the table the patient is asked to move the middle finger sideways (Fig. 9.5). This is a test for the dorsal interossei of middle finger.

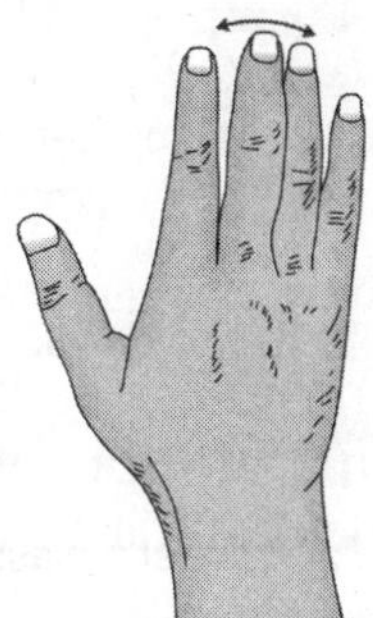

Fig. 9.5: Egawa test

In total clawing median nerve is also injured. Following tests will help to detect the median nerve injury.

Pen test: The patient is unable to touch the pen due to the loss of action of abductor pollicis brevis (Fig. 9.6).

Pointing index or Oschner's clasp test: When both the hands are clasped together, index and middle fingers, fail to flex due to the loss of action of long finger flexors of the index and middle fingers, which are supplied by the median nerve (Fig. 9.7).

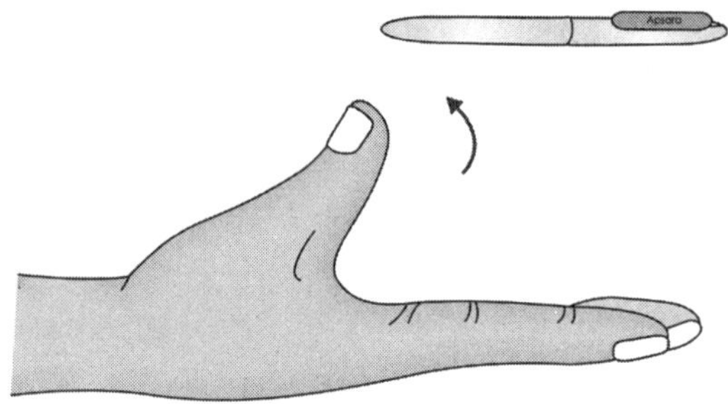

Fig. 9.6: Pen test

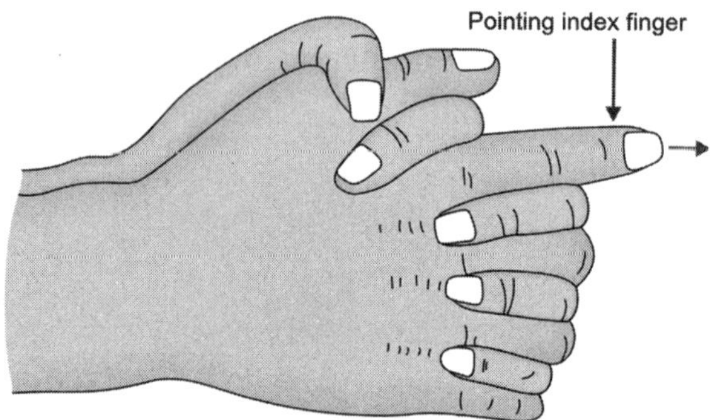

Fig. 9.7: Oschner's clasp test

Benediction test: For the same reason mentioned above, the patient is unable to flex the index and middle finger on lifting the hand. (This is the position a clergyman uses to bless the couple during marriage (Fig. 9.8). Hence, called the benediction test.)

> *Note:* Median nerve supplies the following muscles:
> - *In the forearm:* Pronator teres, flexor carpi radialis, palmaris longus, flexor digitorum superficialis, flexor digitorum profundus, flexor pollicis longus and pronator quadratus.
> - *In the hand:* Abductor and flexor pollicis brevis, opponens pollicis middle and index lumbricals.

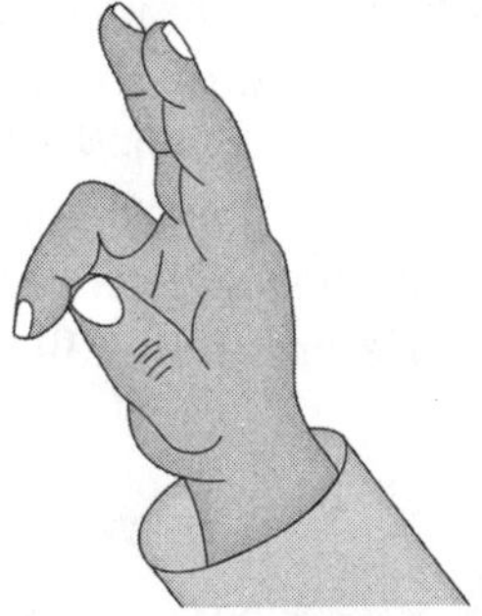

Fig. 9.8: Benediction test

What is ulnar paradox?

The higher the lesion of the median and ulnar nerve injury, the less prominent is the deformity and vice versa. This is because in higher lesions the long finger flexors are paralyzed. The loss of finger flexion makes the deformity look less obvious.

Treatment of Ulnar Nerve Injury

In acute injuries, the treatment is as discussed in the general principles.

For Claw Hand Deformity

Principles of treatment: All the treatment measures aim at blocking the hyperextension at the metacarpophalangeal joint. Once this joint is stabilized, the long extensors will bring about the extension of IP joints. The long finger flexors will help in flexion of the MP joints along with their action of finger and wrist flexion.

Methods of Stabilization of MP Joints

This can be done by the *active method, which involves tendon transfer,* or by *passive method, which involves arthrodesis, capsulodesis or tenodesis.*

Active method: This is by tendon transfers. A neighboring healthy tendon is brought to replace the action of the lost intrinsic. The available normal tendons and the existing local situations dictate the choice of the tendon. *Whichever the tendon chosen, it is passed through the lumbrical canal and is attached to the dorsal digital expansion, which then brings about the action of the lost intrinsics.* Before resorting to tendon transfers, certain criteria are to be followed.

Choice of Surgery

Modified S Bunnell's Operation

When finger flexors are strong, wrist flexors and extensors are strong, and if there is no habitual flexion of the wrist, modified S Bunnell's operation is preferred in which flexor digitorum superficialis of the ring finger is transferred through the lumbrical canal into the dorsal digital expansion.

Riordan's Operation

When flexion of the wrist has become habitual or if there is a flexion contracture of the wrist, a wrist flexor can be spared to overcome the above-mentioned problems. In Riordan's operation, the flexor carpi radialis muscle is removed and transferred with a free tendon graft leaving behind the flexor carpi ulnaris to bring about the wrist flexion.

Brand's Operation

When the finger flexors are weak, the wrist flexors are also weak and when the wrist extensors are strong extensor carpi radialis longus or brevis is transferred by a free tendon graft.

Fowler's Operation

When finger flexors, wrist extensors and wrist flexors are not available for transfer, extensor digitorum longus tendon of the index and little fingers are transferred by the Fowler's technique.

When no muscle is available for transfer and if the joints are supple, capsulodesis of MP joint or tenodesis is done. If the joints are not supple, arthrodesis in functional position is done.

Tardy Ulnar Nerve Palsy

It is late onset ulnar nerve palsy and could be due to the following causes:

- Malunion or nonunion of lateral condyle fracture of humerus.
- Fracture medial epicondyle of humerus.
- Dislocation of elbow.
- Nerve contusions.
- Cubitus valgus.
- Shallow ulnar groove.
- Hypoplasia of humeral trochlea.
- Recurrent subluxation due to inadequate fibrous arch.

Treatment is by anterior transposition of the ulnar nerve.

Entrapment Neuropathy

Entrapment sites: The ulnar nerve could be entrapped in any one of the following sites during its anatomical course:

- Supracondylar process medially.
- Arcade of Stuther's (near medial intermuscular septum).
- Between two heads of flexor carpi ulnaris.
- Guyon's canal.

At a glance: Ulnar nerve injury

- Ulnar nerve root value is C_8T_1.
- Injury causes ulnar clawing.
- Total clawing when median nerve is also affected.
- Froment's sign is a reliable test.
- For quick clinical evaluation after injury, the tip of the little finger is tested for sensation.
- Ulnar paradox—higher the lesion less is the deformity and vice versa.
- Correction is by tendon transfers if all criteria are met.
- If no tendons are available for transfer, MP joint is stabilized by capsulodesis, tenodesis or arthrodesis.
- All surgeries aim at correcting the hyperextension at MP joint.

RADIAL NERVE INJURY

Radial nerve can be entrapped at the following sites (Fig 9.9)

- In the arm—fibrous arch of lateral head of triceps.
- In the forearm—arcade of Frohse.
- At the elbow—radial tunnel syndrome at origin of extensor carpiradialis brevis.
- At the wrist—scar tissue compressing the superficial radial nerve.

Causes for Radial Nerve Injury

The course of the radial nerve and its supply is shown in Fig. 9.9.

General

Metabolic diseases, collagen diseases, malignancies, endogenous or exogenous toxins; thermal, chemical or mechanical trauma, etc. can cause injury to the peripheral nerves.

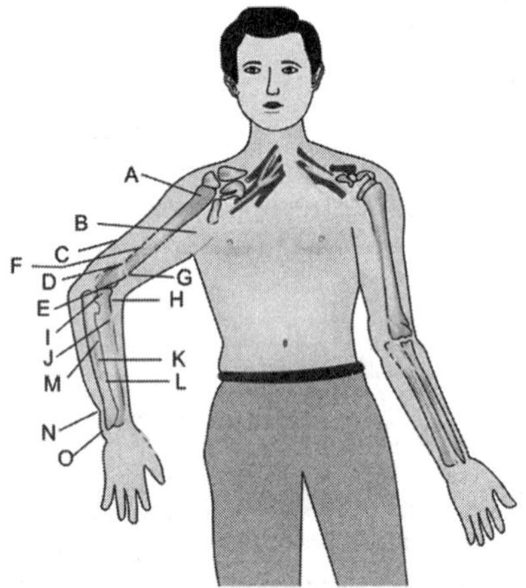

Fig. 9.9: Course of the radial nerve and its supply: (A) Medial head of triceps, (B) Long head of triceps, (C) Lateral head of triceps, (D) Brachioradialis, (E) Extensor carpi radialis longus, (F) Extensor carpiradialis brevis, (G) Anconeus, (H) Supinator, (I) Extensor digitorum longus, (J) Extensor digitorum minimi, (K) Extensor carpi ulnaris, (L) Abductor pollicis longus, (M) Extensor pollicis longus, (N) Extensor pollicis brevis, and (O) Extensor indices

Local

In the axilla
- Aneurysm of the axillary vessels.
- Crutch palsy.

In the shoulder
- Proximal humeral fractures.
- Shoulder dislocation.

In the spiral groove 5's
- Shaft fracture.
- Saturday night palsy (Fig. 9.10).

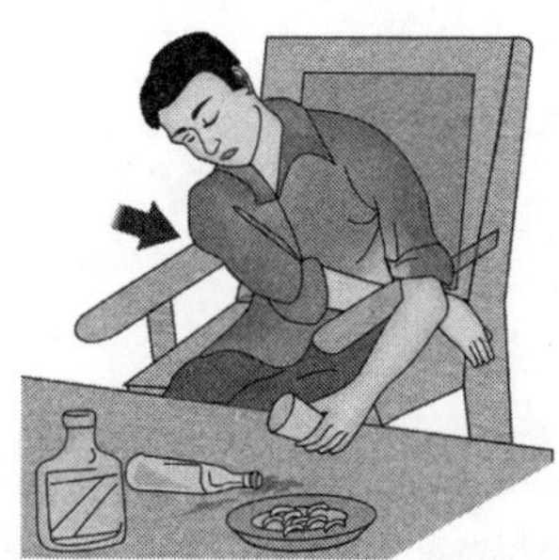

Fig. 9.10: Saturday night palsy (Patient's mistake)

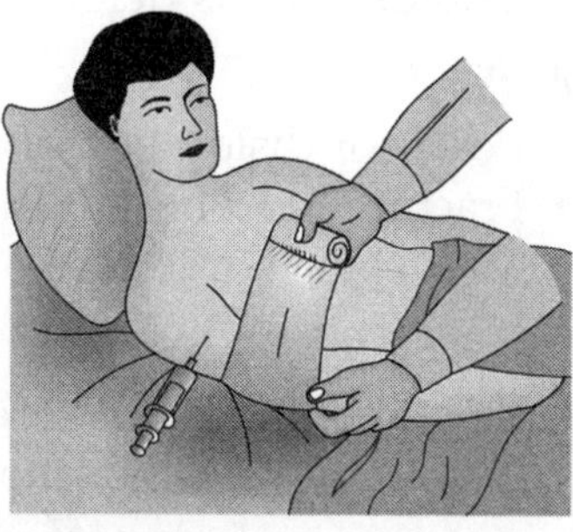

Fig. 9.11: Injection and tourniquet palsy (Doctor's mistake)

- Syringe palsy (Fig. 9.11).
- Surgical positions (Trendelenburg).
- 'S'march's (Esmarch) tourniquet palsy.

Saturday night palsy (Also called weekend palsy)

In this condition, there is compression of the radial nerve between the radiospiral groove and the lateral intermuscular septum.

It is known after an event which typically happens on a Saturday night weekend when in an inebriated condition, a person slumps with his midarm compressed between the arm of the chair and his body.

Did you know about honeymoon palsy?

- You have heard about Saturday night palsy, but have you heard about honeymoon palsy?
- Well, it is sleep palsy and is seen in young couples where a bed partner's head compresses the radial nerve, while resting in the crook of the partner's arms.

Between Spiral Groove and Lateral Epicondyle

- Fracture shaft humerus (Fig. 9.12).
- Supracondylar fracture humerus.
- Lateral epicondyle fracture of the humerus.
- Penetrating and gunshot injuries.
- Cubitus valgus deformity.

At the elbow

- Posterior dislocation of the elbow.
- Fracture head of radius.
- Monteggia's fractures.

Causes in the forearm

- Fracture both bones forearm.
- Penetrating and gunshot injuries.

Levels of lesion

	Features
High: Above spiral groove	Total palsy
Low: Type I *Between:* The spiral groove and the lateral epicondyle	 *Spared:* Elbow extensor ***Lost:* Motor** • Wrist extensor • Thumb extensor • Finger extensors *Sensory:* Dorsum of first web space.
Low: Type II Below the elbow	 *Spared* • Elbow extensor • Wrist extensor *Lost* : Motor • Thumb extensor • Finger extensor *Sensation* first web space

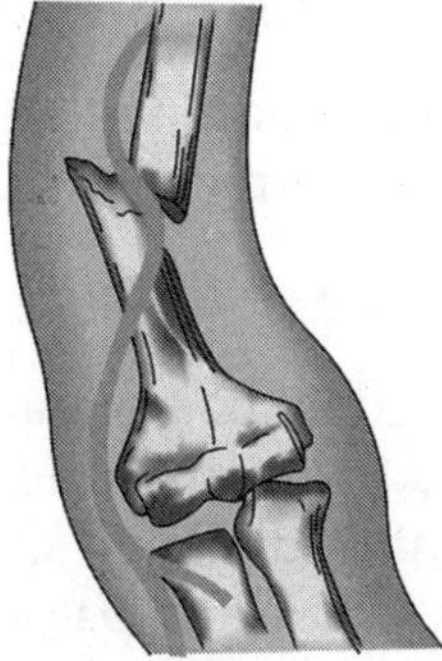

Fig. 9.12: Entrapment of radial nerve in between the fracture fragments of the humerus (nobody's mistake)

Clinical Features

If the lesion is high, the patient will present with wrist drop (Fig. 9.13), thumb drop and finger drop. He will be unable to extend the elbow. If the lesion is low the elbow extension is spared; but the wrist, thumb and the finger extensions are lost, but *the patient can extend the IP joints of the fingers because of the action of the intrinsic muscles of the hand*. Sensation along the posterior surface of the arm and forearm is lost in high lesions and in low lesions the above sensations are spared, but there is loss of sensation over the first dorsal web space.

In acute injuries, it is difficult to evaluate the injury to the radial nerve. In such situations, the Hitchhiker's sign (inability to extend the thumb) is used as the screening test.

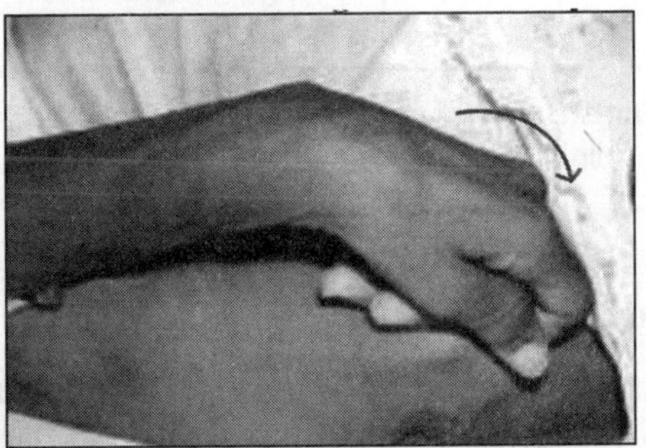

Fig. 9.13: Wrist drop (clinical photo)

Investigations

Radiograph of the injured part and all other investigations mentioned in the general principles are carried out.

Treatment

Early cases: As mentioned in the general principles for closed fractures, conservative treatment is adopted. The patient is put on a cock-up splint or dynamic splints (Figs 9.14A and B). This is followed by active and passive physiotherapy. In failed conservative treatment, operative treatment is considered after a period of 12–18 months.

In open fractures, surgery is the treatment of choice. If the wound is clean, primary nerve repair is done, and if the wound is contaminated, delayed primary or secondary nerve repair is resorted to.

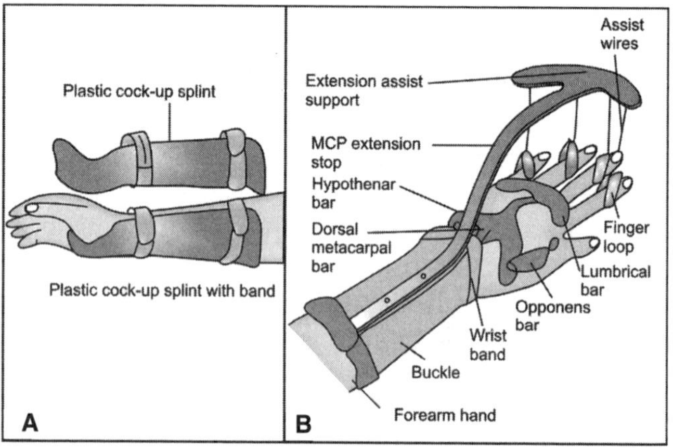

Figs 9.14A and B: Wrist drop splints: (A) Static or cock-up splint, (B) Dynamic splint

Treatment of Late Cases (> 1 year)

Broad principles

Active treatment: If neighboring tendons are intact and if all the criteria for tendon transfers mentioned earlier are met, then tendon transfer is the treatment of choice.

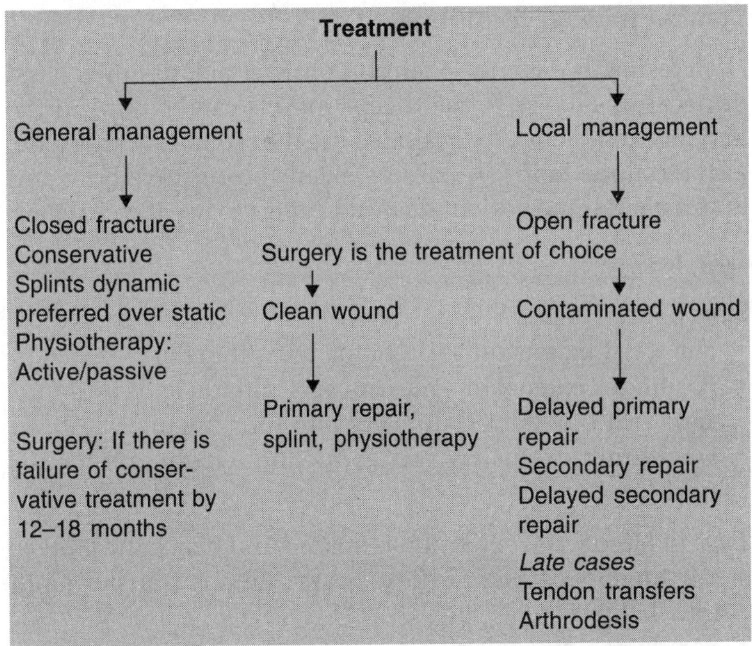

Passive method: If no tendons are available for transfer, then tenodesis or wrist arthrodesis in functional position is preferred.

Choice of tendons in active treatment

From the wrist flexors Flexor carpi ulnaris can be spared. Flexor carpi radialis takes care of the wrist flexion. Palmaris longus is not a very strong wrist flexor and hence can be spared.

From the pronators: Pronator teres can be spared as pronator quadratus takes care of pronation.

From the finger flexors, rarely a flexor digitorum superficialis can be chosen.

Therefore, the tendons chosen for transfer in radial nerve injuries are flexor carpi ulnaris, palmaris longus, pronator teres and rarely flexor digitorum superficialis.

Tendon transfer techniques

High lesion: For elbow extension transfer of latissimus dorsi or pectoralis major to the triceps muscle can be done, if the patient needs active extension to use the crutches. Otherwise, gravity alone helps in passive extension of the elbow and is sufficient if the patient does not prefer to use the crutches.

Low lesions

Type I

- For wrist extension →pronator teres transfer.
- For finger extension →flexor carpi ulnaris split into four slips and transferred dorsally into four fingers.
- For thumb extension and abduction →palmaris longus transfer.

Type II: Here wrist extension is spared and hence the plan is:

- For finger extension →flexor carpi ulnaris transfer (split into 4 slips).
- For thumb extension →palmaris longus transfer.
- For thumb abduction →pronator teres transfer.

Omer's technique: Consists of splitting flexor carpi ulnaris into five slips and transferring into all the five fingers instead of four.

Boye's technique: Uses flexor digitorum superficialis instead of flexor carpi ulnaris to bring about extension of four fingers.

Problems in radial nerve injury

- Wrist drop.
- Thumb drop.
- Finger drop only at MCP joint but extension at IP joint is possible due to action of interossei.
- Sensation over dorsal first web space is lost.
- In high lesions inability to extend the elbow and loss of sensations over posterior surface of arm and forearm are additional problems.

Radial nerve injury at a glance

- Continuation of posterior cord of the brachial plexus.
- Most common peripheral nerve to be injured.
- Most common site of injury is the distal end of humerus.
- Thumb extension test (Hitchhiker's sign) is the screening test.
- In radial nerve injury extension at finger IP joint is still possible.
- For early cases in closed fractures conservative treatment.
- For open fractures operative treatment and repair.
- For late cases, tendon transfers if neighboring tendons are available and if all the criteria are met.
- If no tendons are available, wrist arthrodesis is done in functional position.

Interesting nerve palsies concerning radial nerve

Did you know about handcuff palsy, dog handlers palsy or Cheiralgia paresthetica?

Well, all these are due to compression of the sensory branch of the superficial radial nerve at the level of the distal one-third of the forearm where it pierces the deep fascia and becomes dorsal.

INJURY TO SCIATIC NERVE (Figs 9.15 and 9.16)

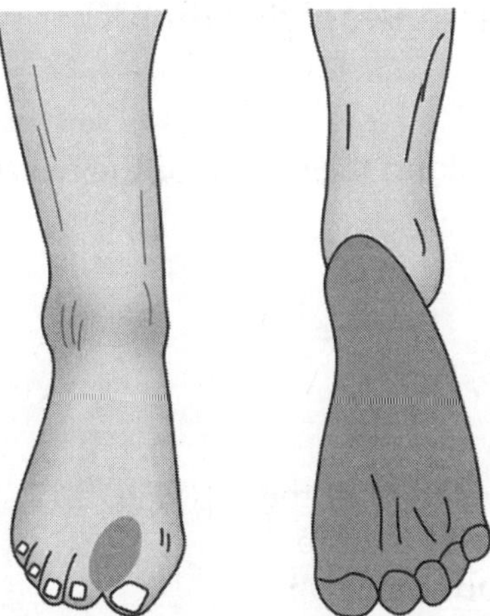

Fig. 9.15: Dorsal web space is supplied by anterior tibial nerve. Sole of the foot is by posterior tibial nerve

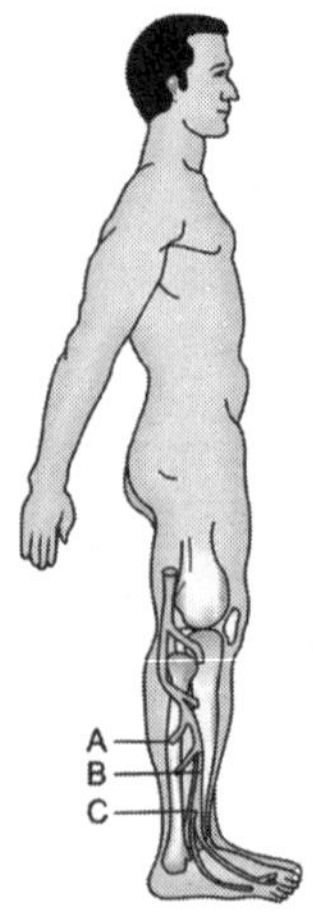

Fig. 9.16: Course of common peroneal (lateral popliteal) nerve: (A) Tibialis anterior, (B) Extensor hallucis longus, (C) Extensor digitorum longus

FOOT-DROP

Causes of Foot-drop

General

Causes have been already mentioned, the important one being leprosy as a cause of foot-drop.

Local

Causes are seen along the course of the nerve.

At the spine
- Spina bifida
- Tumors
- Disk prolapse, etc.

At the hip
- Posterior dislocation of the hip (Fig. 9.17).
- Fractures around the hip.
- Fracture acetabulum.

At the glutei region
Deep intramuscular injections.

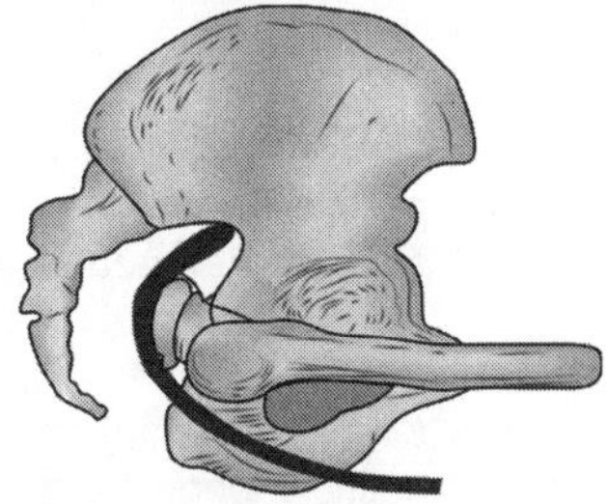

Fig. 9.17: Injury to sciatic nerve due to posterior dislocation of hip joint

At the thigh

- Fracture shaft femur.
- Penetrating injury and gunshot injury.

At the knee (Common causes)

- Forcible inversion of the knee.
- Dislocation of knee.
- Fracture lateral condyle of tibia.
- Lateral meniscal cysts and tumors.
- Dislocation of superior tibiofibular joint.
- Tight plaster casts around the knee.
- Poor padding during traction.
- Surgical damage during application of skeletal traction.
- *Direct injuries*—gunshot injuries, incised and penetrating injuries, etc.

Clinical Features

The resulting deformity following injury to the above nerves is foot-drop (Fig. 9.18). This could either be complete (in sciatic nerve or lateral popliteal nerve injury) or incomplete (injury to either superficial or deep peroneal nerve).

In high lesions, it is a total foot-drop and in low lesions, the foot-drop is usually incomplete. In low type I, the patient cannot dorsiflex and invert the foot but eversion is possible, front of the leg is wasted. In low type II, the patient cannot evert but can dorsiflex and invert the foot. There is wasting of the outer half of the leg. In type I, injury sensation over the

Levels of lesion	
High lesion (Above knee)	**Both tibial nerve and common** peroneal nerve is paralyzed.
Low lesion (Below knee)	*Spared:* Peroneus longus and brevis.
Type I	
Anterior tibial nerve injury	*Lost:* Tibialis anterior, extensor hallucis longus, extensor digitorum longus and peroneus tertius. *Sensation:* Over first web space is lost.
Type II	
Musculocutaneous nerve injury	*Spared:* All the above muscles innervated by anterior tibial nerve. *Lost:* Peroneus longus and brevis. *Sensation:* Over outer leg and foot.

dorsal web space is lost and in type II, injury it is lost over outer leg and foot.

The gait typical of foot-drop is a *high stepping gait.*

Treatment of Early Foot-drop

The lesions show a high incidence of recovery. Hence, conservative treatment with a view to encourage recovery (at least for 1 year) should be carried out.

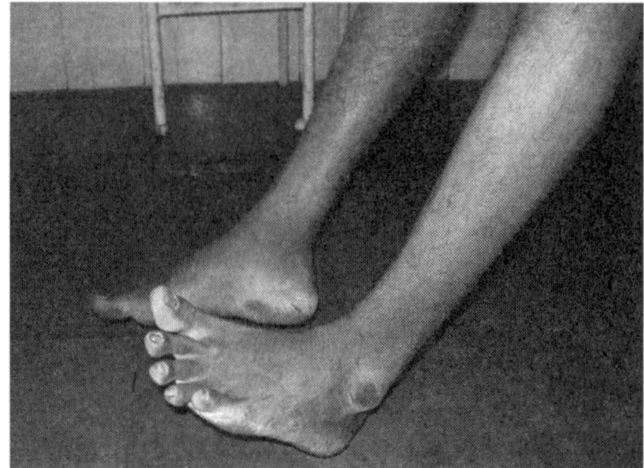

Fig. 9.18: Foot-drop (clinical photo)

Splintage of knee in 20° of flexion and ankle in 90° for nighttime. In the daytime, walking is allowed by using a "Foot-drop appliance".

Foot-drop appliances are of two varieties:

- Dynamic—spring shoe (Fig. 9.19).
- Static—backstop shoe (Fig. 9.20).

Along with the splintage, general treatment to correct the underlying etiology is undertaken. Steroids are also known to help.

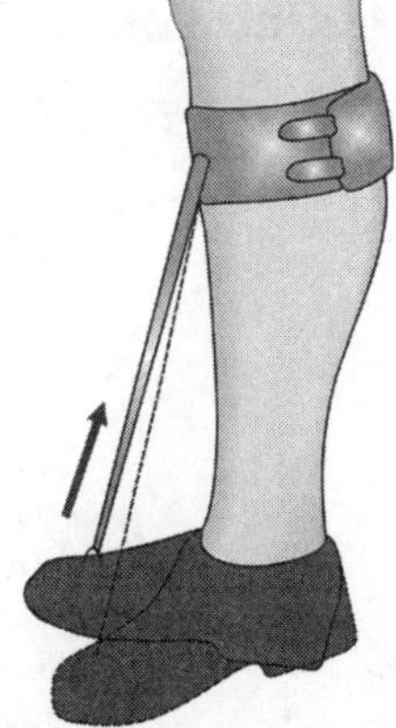

Fig. 9.19: Dynamic foot-drop splint

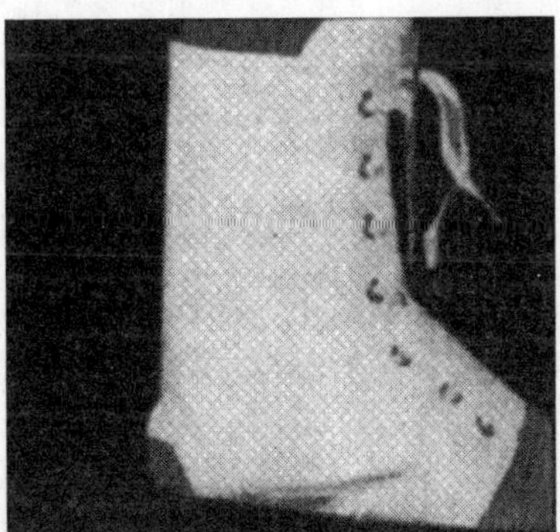

Fig. 9.20: Foot-drop splint (static variety)

Common peroneal nerve stripping is done in leprosy. It is done in a thickened, tender nerve in a tuberculoid case with history of recent paralysis.

Choice of Surgery

- Tendon transfers—for mobile foot-drop.
- Tendo-Achilles lengthening—in fixed equinus.
- Subtalar stabilizing procedure—for fixed varus.
- Triple arthrodesis—for fixed varus at the subtalar joint.

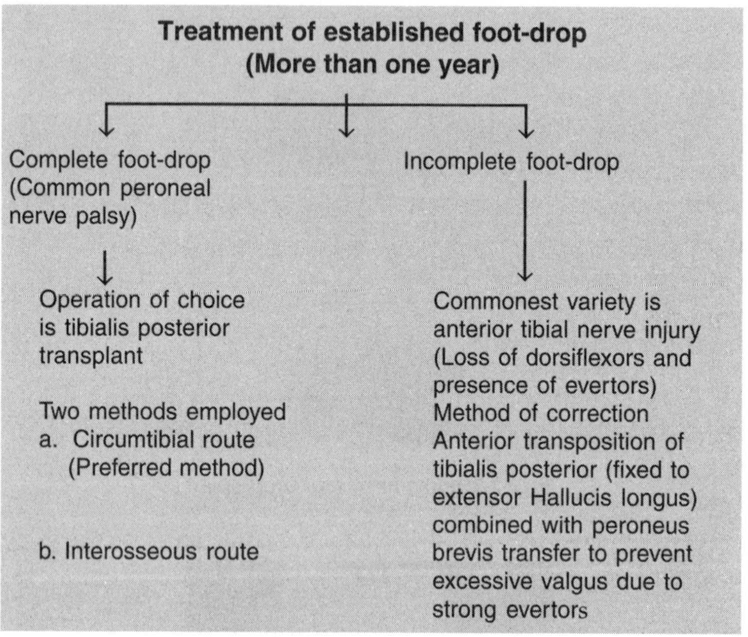

At a glance

- Sciatic nerve is the thickest nerve in the body.
- Common peroneal nerve also called as lateral popliteal nerve is commonly injured at the fibular neck.
- Leprosy is the commonest general cause.
- Foot-drop could be complete or incomplete.
- High stepping gait is characteristic.
- Dynamic foot-drop splint is the mainstay of conservative treatment.
- Conservative treatment is indicated up to one year.
- Tendon transfer for mobile foot-drop contemplated after 1 year.

MERALGIA PARESTHETICA

It is due to compression neuropathy or neuroma of the lateral femoral cutaneous nerve (Fig. 9.21).

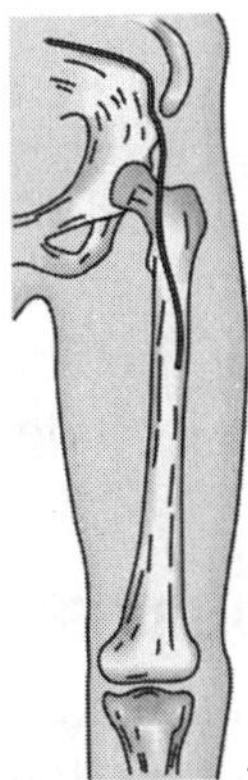

Fig. 9.21: Course of the lateral femoral cutaneous nerve

Types

Idiopathic: Here, the exact cause is unknown.

Spontaneous: This is due to mechanical compression anywhere throughout the course of the nerve. The common site of injury is at the exit of the nerve at the pelvis.

Iatrogenic: This is commonly seen after orthopedic surgeries like anterior iliac crest bone grafting and anterior pelvic procedures and prone positioning for surgeries.

Clinical Features

This is characterized by pain, numbness and paresthesia along the anterolateral aspect of the thigh.

Diagnostic Test

If there is relief of pain and paresthesia after injecting local anesthetic, the diagnosis is clinched.

Treatment

Conservative

Idiopathic type: Improves by removal of the compressive agents, nonsteroidal anti-inflammatory drugs and local steroid injection.

Iatrogenic type: Care should be exercised during pelvic surgery.

Operative

If pain persists in spite of the above treatment, surgery is indicated. The procedures include neurolysis or transection of the nerves.

BRACHIAL PLEXUS INJURIES

Everything about brachial plexus is complex, its anatomy (Fig.9.22), mode of injury, the diagnosis, management and prognosis. It is a narrowing experience for both the patient and the surgeon. Among the more famous causes of brachial plexus, injury is the birth injury in children and bike injury in adults.

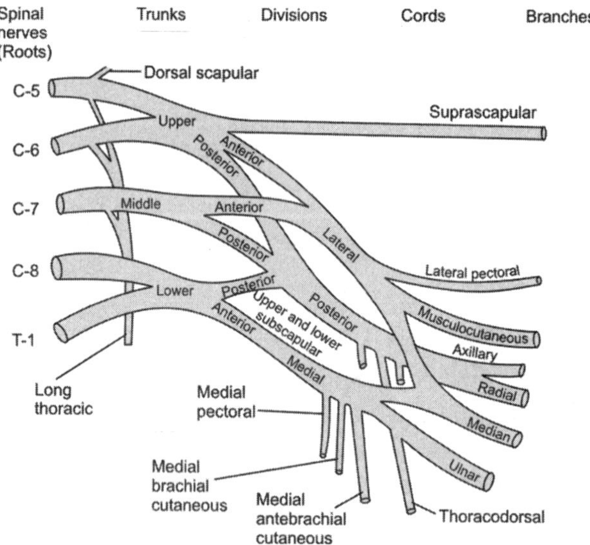

Fig. 9.22: The normal anatomy of brachial plexus

Causes

Brachial plexus injuries (Figs 9.23A and B) could be

Closed: Here the injury could be due to birth trauma or bike trauma as mentioned above.

Open: It is a rare injury and could be due to penetrating or gun-shot injuries.

> *Note:* Other fewer important causes of brachial plexus injuries:
> - Traction injuries
> - Tumor removal
> - Abnormal pressures due to faculty postures
> - Post irradiation scenario
> - Surgical excision of cervical ribs
> - Shoulder dislocations.

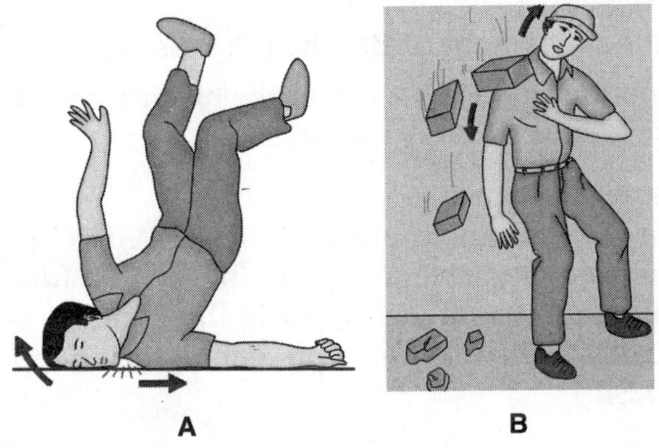

Figs 9.23 A and B: Mechanism of brachial plexus injury

TYPES OF LESIONS

Supraclavicular Lesion

Pre-ganglionic Lesion

This is an unfortunate situation wherein the nerve roots are avulsed from the spinal cord. The cause could be either birth or bike trauma as mentioned earlier. The characteristic feature of this lesion is the presence of Horner's syndrome (Fig. 9.24).

Interesting facts

About Horner's syndrome

What constitutes a Horner's syndrome? (All P's)

- Ptosis of the eyelid.
- Pupils, which are small and constricted.
- Protrusion of the eyeball, which is slight.
- Pain even at rest.
- Positive sensory action potentials.
- Poor prognosis.

Postganglionic Lesions

Here there is no Horner's syndrome. The prognosis is slightly better than the preganglionic lesion. A positive Tinel's sign may be elicited in this lesion.

Clinical Assessment of Brachial Plexus Injury

It is important to assess whether the brachial plexus injury is preganglionic or postganglionic.

In preganglionic lesions

- Horner's syndrome is present (Fig. 9.24A).
- The patient is unable to elevate the scapula (due to the disruption in the nerve supply to the Rhomboids and L scapulae). The patient may present with flail upper limb (Fig 9.24B).

In postganglionic lesions

- No Horner's syndrome.
- The patient is able to elevate the scapula.
- Tinel's sign is present in the later stages. (Tapping above the clavicle, produces tingling sensation in the anesthetic limb.)

Investigations

These are less reliable than the clinical tests. However, X-ray to rule out neck fractures, CT scan to study the cross-section anatomy, MRI to study the soft tissue damages, myelogram (shows meningocele in avulsion, but hazardous) and

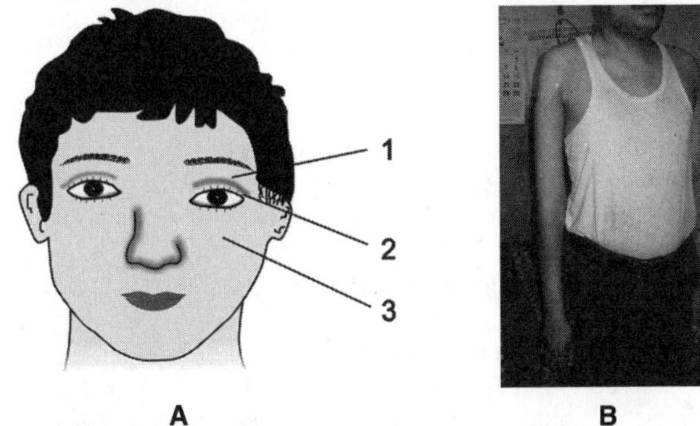

Figs 9.24A and B: Features of Horner's syndrome: (A) (1) Drooping of the eyelid, (2) Constricted pupil, (3) Absence of sweating in the surrounding skin, (B) Flail upper limb (clinical photo)

electrical studies are some of the investigations which give useful information during a brachial plexus injury.

The electrodiagnostic tests include EMG, nerve conduction study, SEP (somatosensoryevoked potential), percutaneous electrical stimulation, etc. EMG is by far the most reliable and effective test, which successfully identifies the roots, involved.

Treatment

During the initial stages

- *Splinting*
  - *For complete paralysis:* A flail arm splint (FAS) designed by Framton is advised.
  - *For incomplete lesions:* Here splints with necessary modifications as per the situations can be used.

During the Later Stages

Measures to strengthen the muscles: If there are movements, efforts are made to strengthen the muscles by repeated self-resistive exercises, PNF techniques, etc.

Quick facts

About FAS

- It immobilizes the shoulder in abduction.
- It prevents glenohumeral joint subluxation.
- It permits five different positions of the elbow.
- It provides a platform for the forearm on which split hook, etc. can be applied.
- It can be operated through a cable to the shoulder strap attached to the opposite normal limb.
- It is cosmetically acceptable.
- For pain control, TENS is best suited.
- To prevent contractures and deformities, a careful passive ROM exercises under suitable guidance is recommended.

Re-education of the muscles: This is done by encouraging movements of the shoulder, percutaneous electrical stimulation, stimulating techniques like icing, brushing, etc.

Modifying: The splints and dynamizing it helps.

TENS to control pain.

After 2 years, reconstructive surgeries are planned for the residual paralysis and deformities.

Surgical Measures

Acute phases: In pre-ganglionic lesions wherein the roots have avulsed from the cord, surgical exploration serves no purpose. However, suture or nerve grafting can be considered in postganglionic lesions.

Late stages (> 2 years): Reconstructive surgeries are planned after 2 years when the recovery can no longer take place. Surgeries are planned according to the residual paralysis.

- *For shoulder function:* Trapezius transfer to the neck of the humerus to improve abduction is advised.
- Arthrodesis of the shoulder is done in functional position.
- *For elbow function:* Steindler's flexorplasty (transfer of latissimus dorsi or pectoralis major to biceps).

- *For wrist and finger extension:* After the surgery, the patient is put on a detailed regime for re-educating the transplanted muscle.

ERB'S PALSY

This is due to injury to the C_5 nerve root and rarely the C_6 nerve root is injured. It occurs either very early in life due to birth trauma (obstetric palsy, due to faulty application of forceps) or in young adults due to bike trauma (Fig. 9.25).

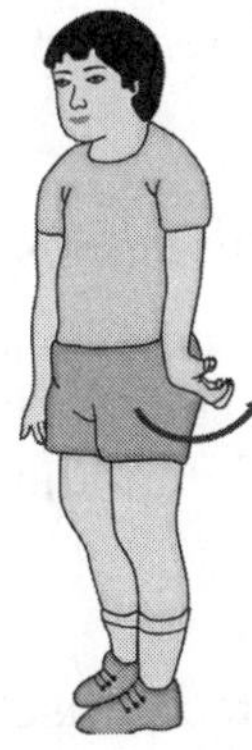

Fig. 9.25: Waiter's or Porter's tip position in Erb's palsy

Effects of the Injury

At the shoulder here, there is paralysis of the deltoid, rhomboids, supra- and infraspinatus and teres minor muscles. This results in the loss of shoulder abduction and external rotation.

At the elbow, biceps and brachialis muscles are paralyzed. This results in loss of flexion of the elbow joint.

At the forearm: Supinator, muscles are paralyzed resulting in loss of supination of the forearm.

The combined effect of the injury is an arm hanging loosely by the side of the trunk. The shoulder is internally rotated, the elbow is in extension, the forearm is pronated and the wrist is in flexion. This characteristic posture is popularly known as *Policeman or Waiter's tip.*

Apart from this, there may be sensory loss on the outer aspects of the arm and forearm both in the front and back.

Management

Splinting

This is done by using an abduction or aeroplane splint. The shoulder is maintained in abduction and external rotation, elbow in 90° of flexion, forearm in supination and wrist in extension.

Measures to Prevent Contractures

A full range of passive movements to the affected joints helps prevent the contractures. This is a home treatment program and should be taught to the mother.

Electrical

Stimulation of the affected muscles by using bilaterally symmetrical PNF stimulus helps to activate them.

Surgery

This is rarely indicated as most of the cases recover spontaneously with the above treatment. Some of the recommended surgical measures are:

- Exploration and repair of the nerve roots.
- Tendon transfers to improve abduction and external rotation of the shoulder.
- Release of soft tissue contractures.
- De-rotation osteotomy for the rotational deformity.

KLUMPKE'S PARALYSIS

This is also due to either a birth trauma or a bike trauma (Fig. 9.26).

The C_8T_1 nerve roots are involved and there will be paralysis of the wrist flexors, finger flexors and intrinsic muscles of the hand. This results in a clawhand deformity. The clinical features and management are dicussed in the section on ulnar and median nerve injuries.

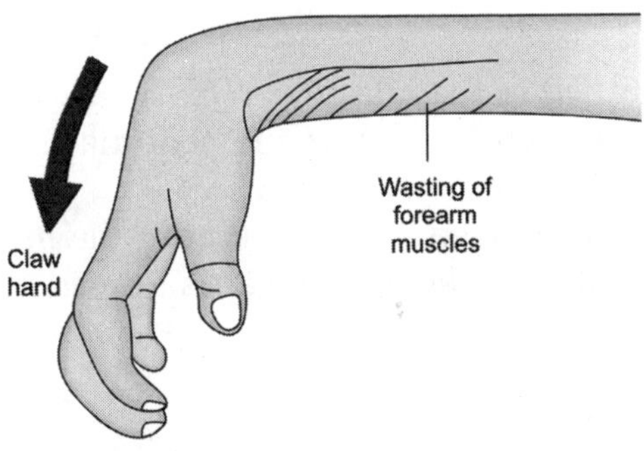

Fig. 9.26: Klumpke's paralysis

AXILLARY NERVE INJURY

Relevant Anatomy

It takes origin from the posterior cord of the brachial plexus and winds round the lower border of the subscapularis. It goes through the quadrangular space and lies medial to the surgical neck of the humerus and divides into anterior and posterior branches. The anterior branch winds around the surgical neck of the humerus and supplies the deltoid muscle except the lower half. Posterior branch supplies the teres minor, lower half of the deltoid and ends as a cutaneous nerve that supplies the lower half of the deltoid region.

Clinical Features

Wasting of the deltoid muscle, regiment badge anesthesia, inability of the patient to abduct the shoulder are some of the classical features.

Treatment

Treatment is essentially conservative management followed by physiotherapy and exercises.

INJURY TO THE LONG THORACIC NERVE (Winging of the Scapula)

Highlights

- It is also called as scapula alta.
- Here the medial border of the scapula is positioned laterally and posteriorly.
- It is called as winged scapula because the inferior angle of the scapula protrudes backwards instead of lying flat.

Causes

- Weakness of the serratus anterior muscles.
- Impingement of the long thoracic nerve.
- Damaged trapezius muscle or denervation of its nerve supply.
- This may be due to injury to the above structures due to repetitive lifting, fall on the shoulders, sports injuries, brachial plexus neuropathies, iatrogenic division of the long thoracic nerve, severe traumatic depression of the shoulder, fascioscapulohumeral dystrophy, fall from the bike, etc.

Relevant Clinical Findings

- Classical winged deformity (Fig. 9.27).
- On pushing against the wall the scapula stands out prominently.
- There may be difficulty in lifting the arm above the head.

Treatment

- *Conservative treatment* consists of physiotherapy, exercises and shoulder rehabilitation.

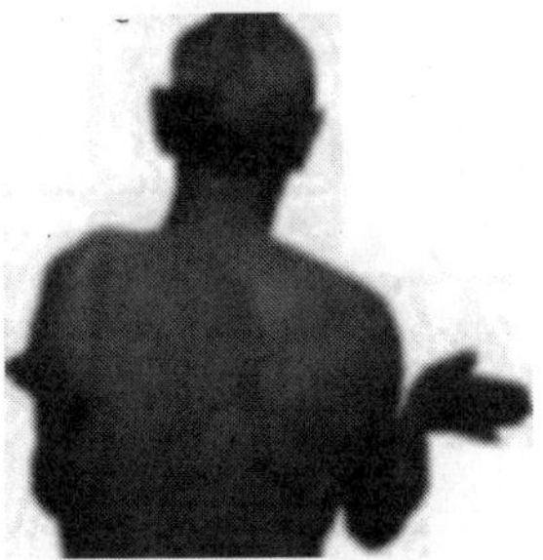

Fig. 9.27: Winging of the scapula (clinical photo)

- *Surgical treatment* is recommended in resistant cases. The recommended procedures are pectoralis major muscle transfer in isolated serratus anterior palsy or scapulodesis in failed transfers.

Index

Acetabular fractures 24
Acetabulum fractures 8
Advantages 146
After reduction 52
Aims of treatment 85
Allen's classification of cervical spine fractures 116
Allis method 55
Anderson and D'olonzo's classification 129
Anterior dislocation of the hip 63
Anteroposterior radiograph lines 31
At the accident site 125
At the hospital 125
Avascular necrosis 97
Axillary nerve injury 181

Based on fracture characters 80
Bedsore management 144
Before reduction 51
Between spiral groove and lateral epicondyle 162
Bigelow's method 55
Both-column fractures 38
Bowel program 145
Brachial plexus injuries 174
Brand's operation 158
Broad classification 79
Broad treatment plans as per garden's classification 86
Burst fracture of C1 128

Cardinal points in internal fixation 90
Cauda equina syndrome 147
Causatively 79
Causes for radial nerve injury 160
Causes of foot-drop 168
Causes of ulnar nerve injury 151
Central dislocation of hip 69
Chance fracture (Seatbelt injury) 131
Chest physiotherapy 23
Choice of an implant 101
Choice of surgery 158, 172
Choices of implants for internal fixation 89
Classical Watson-Jones method 56
Classification: Judet's types 69
Claw hand 153
Clinical assessment 141
Clinical assessment of brachial plexus injury 176
Clinical classification of neurological damage 139
Clinical presentation 39
Clinical significance of vascular anatomy 45
Complications of internal fixation 91
Concussion 117
Conservative 174
Conservative measures 20, 23
CT scan 11, 31

Delayed complications 68
Delbet's classification in children 80
Diagnostic test 173
Double breaks in the pelvic ring 8
During the initial stages 177
During the later stages 177

Effects of the injury 179

Electrical 180
Entrapment neuropathy 159
Epidemiology 25
Epstein's classification 64
Erb's palsy 179

Fixation choices 136
Flexion distraction injury 131
Foot-drop 168
For claw hand deformity 157
For ulnar nerve injury 153
Fowler's operation 158
Fracture neck of femur 75
Fracture of individual bones without a break in the pelvic ring 8
Fracture pelvis 3
Fractures affecting the integrity of the pelvic ring 7
Fractures not affecting the integrity of the pelvic ring 6

General causes 151
Goal of treatment 54

Hangman's fracture 129
Hemireplacement arthroplasty 95
Hemorrhage 16
Highlights 182
History 4

Incidence of spine injuries 113
Indications for open reduction 59
Individual cervical fracture of interest 128
Injection therapy 21
Injuries around the hip joint dislocations and fracture dislocations 44
Injuries around the hip—fractures of neck femur 75
Injuries of lower urinary tract 17
Injuries of the cervical spine 113
Injuries of the coccyx and ribs 19
Injury to sciatic nerve 167
Injury to the coccyx 19
Injury to the long thoracic nerve (Winging of the scapula) 182

Judet and Letournel classifications 27

Key and Conwell's classification 8
Klumpke's paralysis 180

LMN type (Autonomous bladder) 143
Local causes 151

Managing bedsores 145
McAfee's classification—3-column classification 130
Measures to prevent contractures 180
Meralgia paresthetica 173
Methods of closed reduction 54
Methods of reduction 101
Methods of stabilization of MP joints 157
Methods of treatment 61
Methods: ABCDS method of reduction 66
Meyer's muscle pedicle graft 91
Modified Magerl classification (ao/ASIF) 132
Modified s Bunnell's operation 158

Nerve root involvement 118
Nonunion 92

Odontoid process fracture 129
Open reduction option 101
Operative 174
Osteotomy 94
Other complications 17
Other examinations 123
Other injuries 17

Paralyzed bladder 143
Pathology 139
Pathophysiology 26
Pelvic injuries 3
Peripheral nerve injury 151
Physiotherapy management 20
Pipkin types 50
Posterior hip dislocations 48
Postganglionic lesions 176
Postoperative treatment 60
Postreduction protocol 58, 68
Pre-ganglionic lesion 175
Preventing bedsores 144
Principles of treatment 23
Procedure of internal fixation 89
Prognosis in spinal cord injuries 149

Radial nerve injury 160
Radiological assessment of the acetabular fracture 31
Reduce the fracture before fixing it is the mantra 101
Relevant anatomy 24, 181
Relevant clinical findings 182
Rib fractures 21
Riordan's operation 158
Rotary subluxation of C1 or C2 129

Single break in the pelvic ring 8
Spinal cord injury 139
Spinal injuries 109
Splinting 180
Stability of the pelvis 3
Stable burst fractures 131
Stable pelvic fracture 4
Stimson's gravity method 57
Structural classification 79
Supraclavicular lesion 175
Surgery 180
Surgical approaches 42
Surgical excision of the coccyx 21
Surgical measures 178
Surgical treatment 126

Tardy ulnar nerve palsy 159
Technique of open reduction 59
Thompson and Epstein classifications 49
Thoracic and Lumbosacral spine injuries 130
Thromboembolism 92
Tile's classification 9
Total hip replacement 96
Translational injuries 132
Transverse fractures 29, 35
Treatment methods 15, 125
Treatment of early foot-drop 170
Treatment of late cases (> 1 year) 164
Treatment of ulnar nerve injury 157
Trochanteric fracture 98
T-type fractures 37
Type I dislocation 54
Type V posterior fracture dislocations 60
Types of lesions 175
Types of neck fractures 75

Ulnar nerve injury 151
UMN type (Automatic bladder) 143
Unstable burst fractures 131
Unstable pelvic fracture 4
Upper or proximal femoral fractures 75

Vascular anatomy and its significance 77
Vital steps 122

Wedge compression 130

Clinical Notes

Clinical Notes